Prepper's Emergency
Medical Manual

How to Be the Doctor When No Doctor is Around

Henry Holcomb CHES

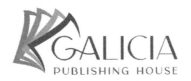

Published by: Galicia Publishing House

Support@BarberryBooks.com

Design & Cover by Olivia O'Neal

First Edition

Contents

Dedication and Foreword

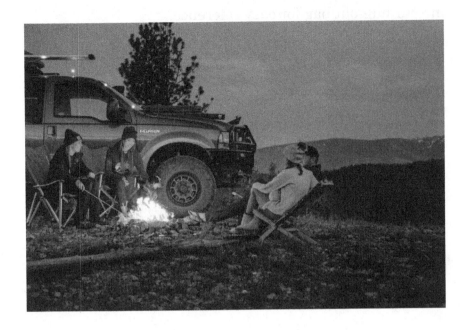

First, I must thank my darling wife. She has put up with my prepping habit, even at the expense of losing nearly all of the storage space in our lovely suburban home. She understands me more than any other human on this Earth. I would be devastated if I were to ever lose her. I know you must feel the same about someone, too. This is why we prepare for the worst and hope for the best.

Also, I thank you, the reader. Thank you for purchasing this book. If you have not already done so, I would recommend buying this in its printed version rather than an eBook so that you can keep it on your stockpile shelf or in your bug-out bag for easy reference.

Please be aware that this is in no way a medical textbook. I am not a doctor, personally, but I believe that everyone, even non-doctors, should know this medical information for the absolute worst-case scenario. There may not always be a doctor around to treat you and your loved ones. It may be all up to you to save them.

Hopefully, this book will help when and if that day ever comes.

Introduction

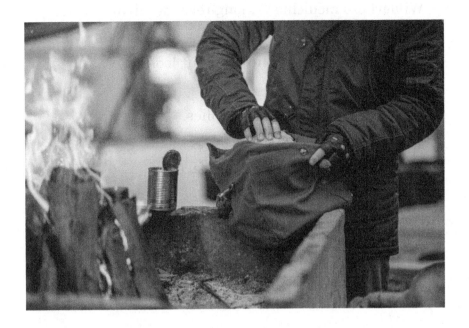

We've been dealing with a terrifying reality since 2020. The COVID-19 pandemic has swept the world and caused many people to start worrying about how they would take care of themselves in the event of a disaster or SHTF event. But what exactly is an SHTF event, and what kind of disasters might take medical personnel out of the picture?

What You Will Learn

In this book, we'll cover all of those questions and many

other topics, including:

Wilderness medicine vs. long-term survival.

How to stockpile supplies without looking crazy.

How to get bulk medical supplies.

Likely medical issues you will face.

How to gain knowledge of medical situations.

How to triage patients and decide who gets treated first.

Basic first aid procedures and CPR treatments.

Definitions of standard medical terms

How to deal with special long-term conditions like diabetes and heart disease.

How to stay safe while providing medical care, including how to get the patient out of a dangerous situation, transporting patients, how to deal with blood and how to deal with contagions, among other things.

Frequently asked questions or dos and don'ts with emergency medicine.

How to deal with the dead.

How to deal with severed body parts like fingers, tones, arms, and legs - we won't be able to reattach them.

Mainly, well focus on medicines and medical necessities a successful prepper needs to survive another pandemic or emergency. These will include common drugs such as antacids, antibiotics, bee sting remedies, cold and flu medicines, and diarrhea, as well as herbal remedies for those same conditions.

We'll also cover how to deal with other emergencies like gunshots, electrocution, radiation exposure, heart attacks, and anaphylactic shock.

What exactly is an SHTF event?

"SHTF" stands for "shit (or stuff) hits the fan." When we talk about these events, we're talking about events like the COVID-19 pandemic or other events that could make it difficult for doctors and emergency personnel to provide medical care, such as:

Major natural disasters

World wars

Nuclear attacks

EMP (electromagnetic pulse)

Economic collapse

Yellowstone eruption

Nationwide martial law

Global warming

Nuclear meltdown

Grid-down event

Megadrought

Food crisis

Technological disaster

Asteroids hitting earth

Cyberattack

Critical power failure

Of these different scenarios, the ones most likely to happen are major natural disasters, pandemics or localized epidemics, solar flares, the full-scale collapse of the power grid, nuclear attacks, and world wars.

Ok, now that I've started making you paranoid, let me reassure you that the purpose of this book is not to make you paranoid, but to make you aware of the different situations that could happen and tell you how to prepare for them when they do. In the next section, we'll talk about how to start and where to start with medical prepping.

How to Start with Medical Prepping

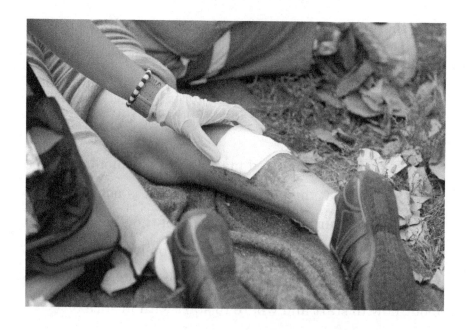

When you're preparing for an SHTF event, you need to know how to start and where to start with medical prepping. Start by deciding how much medication to store for emergencies. When you are storing medicines for emergencies, it is hard to come up with one amount that will work for everyone. Consider the worst-case scenario and determine how much medication you'll need to adequately care for your needs, then stock a little extra to store.

Many medications can still be used after the expiration date. However, fresh medications are better. Therefore, you should only purchase drugs in reasonable amounts. Overstocking will waste medication and may not be the best way to use your money. Some people restock their supplies every few years and get rid of the old medication, so they can keep a fresh supply.

It's reasonable to stock enough over-the-counter medications to last a year or two. Prescription medications are more difficult to obtain, and you may be lucky to have one or two months as a backup supply.

Plan for Your Family Members' Unique Needs

Before you stock your prepper supplies, think about the unique needs of all family members. Consider the following questions:

Are any family members allergic to any medications?

Do you need to have infant or child forms of certain drugs?

Does anyone have unique needs because of a chronic

medical condition?

Does anyone have seasonal allergies?

Does anyone have problems with pain management?

Stock appropriately for people who will use the medication. Keep a supply on hand for everyday needs, not just for emergencies.

Ideal Storage Conditions for Medications

In general, medications are stored best in a cool, dry, dark location in the original unopened packaging. The bathroom medicine cabinet isn't the best place to store your medications because of the heat and humidity. Store all medications away from children.

Drug interactions are a major concern. Some addicts can be identified easily, but others you may never suspect. Consider storing prescription medications in a locked, safe or well-hidden location to protect both the drug seeker and your critical medications.

Keeping fresh medications on hand is always a good

idea. It may, however, be important to understand the actual shelf-life in case you need to use older medications during a crisis.

According to Cynthia Koelker, MD, who wrote "Armageddon Medicine," many drugs retain 90% of their potency for at least five years after expiration dates on the label. There will be a gradual loss of potency over time. The medication is probably safe to consume if the appearance and color of the pills have not changed. Storage temperature and packaging greatly affect shelf-life. Liquid preparations aren't as stable as tablets and capsules and generally have a shorter usable shelf-life.

The Best Way to Stockpile Prescription Medications

It's possible that your supply of prescription medications may be interrupted when disaster strikes. If you take medications for a chronic medical condition, it would be wise to plan in advance to take care of your needs.

You should strive to improve your health in order to reduce your dependence on prescription medications.

Meanwhile, stock up on enough medications to last you through a crisis.

Prepare a backup supply of critical prescription medications with your physician. Discuss your concerns with them. Always follow their advice and make sure your supplies are rotated.

Medical providers won't give you any type of controlled substance (drugs that may cause physical or mental dependence) for emergency preparedness. Don't bother asking. Medical providers are frequently given free samples of drugs by drug companies. If he or she gives you a few samples, make sure you keep filling your prescription on schedule. You can easily get a 30-60 day backup supply like this.

Your prescription will usually be refilled every 25 days by your insurance company. By the end of a year, if you pick up your prescription on time at 25 days, you will have a backup supply of 60 days. Your medication may be available from a mail-order pharmacy for a 90-day supply. Refill it as soon as possible.

You can also ask your doctor to give you a prescription for an extra month that you can pay for in cash at your local pharmacy. You may be able to avoid limitations imposed by your health insurance by doing this.

Creating the Perfect Prepper Medication Stockpile

Here's how you can build a stockpile of everyday medications.

Go through the medications you currently have and get rid of outdated drugs.

Write down all the medications your family may need and the amount of each. Include special formulations for babies and the elderly.

Any special needs of family members should be discussed with your healthcare provider. Examine the possibility of obtaining additional prescription medications for chronic conditions or storing antibiotics in case of an emergency.

Choose a place to store your medications. Opened bottles should be stored in a medicine cabinet or with first aid supplies and backup supplies in a cool, dry, dark, and secure place.

Buy a fresh supply of over-the-counter medications at your local pharmacy or online.

Likely Issues You Will Face

Assuming that you have collected the right medical supplies and you are in a position to use them, there are many medical issues you should expect to come your way. When stocking up your medical supplies, you may want to check out some of these issues and find solutions.

Dosage of Drugs

One of the major challenges you may face in case we come to a point where your stockpile finds work is the dosage. In most cases, the drugs sold over the counter would not be sold with a prescription but should be labeled with dosage instructions.

With prescription medication, it is the prescription that provides the right dosages. In a situation where you can't access a doctor or a pharmacy, you should have an idea of how the drug should be administered. To prevent having to come to such a situation, keep a dedicated record book in your medical supplies room. In the book, note down every drug you purchase, the way it is administered, and the right dosage. At the moment (before the SHFT emergency), you can easily get most of the necessary information by consulting a pharmacist or a friend doctor. Some of the information may even be available online. In an SHFT event, you may not even have access to the internet.

Drug Expiration

The other issue you are likely to encounter is drug expiration. Some drugs that are stocked may last only a few days on the shelf. This may lead to having some drugs on your shelf that are already expired. However, as already mentioned in the sections above, drugs can be used even after expiration in case you are in a life and death situation. Experts have proven that drugs retain up to 90% of their active components even after expiry. In other words, the drugs piled up can be stored for up to a year.

Storage Problems

There are some types of medications that can only be stored in a cool environment, such as the refrigerator. In a situation where there is a shift in living style, chances are that you may not have a fridge around. In some situations, there may even not be an electricity supply to power refrigerators. In such a situation, you should have alternative ways of handling your medical supplies to keep them cool.

One of the ways of keeping things cool even in a hot environment is by storing them in clay pots with some water. Clay pots are amazing coolants that can help keep drugs that need refrigeration in a usable state for some time. The ideal scenario would be filling the pot with water to the halfway mark. Seal the necessary drugs in a water-proof bag and drop them in the water. This way, the drugs will remain cool for long.

You may also use other options, such as creating storage spaces on concrete floors. We all know that concrete remains relatively cool indoors and can help keep certain things cool. Keeping the supplies on a cold floor may help in improving its lifespan.

With all that said, refrigeration cannot be completely replaced by natural alternatives. If you ever find yourself in a situation where you have to use natural refrigeration, remember that it can only provide supplementary help. This may mean that it helps ensure that the drugs are usable for a few days.

How to Obtain Bulk Medical Supplies

In addition to food and other things, you'll need bulk medical supplies. What if the supplies run out in your first aid kit or emergency stockpile? You can obtain some bulk medical supplies from Amazon. Otherwise, you may have to contact a bulk medical supply company for items like medical face masks, sanitizing and disinfecting wipes, protective and sanitary head coverings, oxygen machines and filtration systems, medical pipettes, and viral and bacterial test kits.

Medicines and Medical Necessities

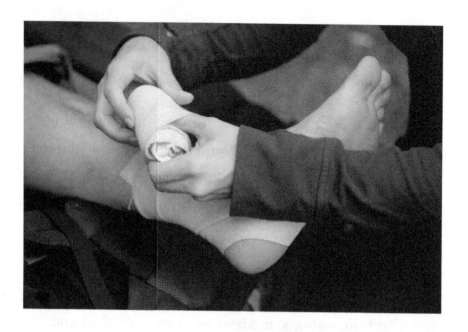

As the world navigates through the phase of COVID-19, people are starting to realize that pandemics could happen. Another emergency or pandemic will happen sooner or later. Emergencies can occur at any time, be it medical, natural, or political. It is necessary for every person to find a way of dealing with these emergencies. In this section, we will be looking at some of the supplies you will need for medical preparedness in case of another SHFT event that would destabilize your normal lifestyle.

The Best Over-the-Counter Medications to Stockpile

It's easier and less expensive to stock your supplies with useful over-the-counter medications. Carefully consider your family's needs and include the meds they regularly use. The following medications are a good place to start:

Ibuprofen (Motrin, Advil)

Ibuprofen treats both pain and inflammation. It's commonly used to relieve headaches, earaches, sore throats, sinus pain, muscle strains, menstrual cramps, arthritis pain, and back pain. It's also good for reducing fevers.

When it's used in conjunction with acetaminophen (Tylenol), it's very good at relieving severe pain. People who have teeth pulled can use ibuprofen and acetaminophen to relieve the pain instead of using narcotics, which can be addictive.

Naproxen (Aleve)

Naproxen is a non-steroidal anti-inflammatory drug.

Like ibuprofen, It works well for relieving pain, fever, and inflammation. Unlike Ibuprofen, it can last up to 12 hours. It could be a good one to stock if some of your family members prefer it.

Aspirin (Bayer, Ecotrin)

Aspirin can reduce fever, control pain, and reduce swelling and inflammation. It's also used as a blood thinner in low doses to prevent heart attacks, strokes, and blood clots. Children younger than 12 should not take this medication if they have a fever because of the risk of Reye's syndrome.

Acetaminophen (Tylenol)

Acetaminophen is the only over-the-counter pain reliever that is not an anti-inflammatory drug. It won't irritate the stomach like ibuprofen, aspirin, or naproxen. It's effective for both pain relief and fever reduction. It may be good for family members who can't take ibuprofen.

Diphenhydramine (Benadryl)

Diphenhydramine is an inexpensive antihistamine. It's used to relieve symptoms from respiratory infections, hay fever, and allergies. It's also helpful for treating hives, itching, nausea, anxiety, and insomnia.

Loperamide (Imodium)

This drug is used to control diarrhea and relieve intestinal cramping. Diarrhea can quickly cause dehydration, which makes this medication a good choice to keep in stock.

Polyethylene Glycol 3350 (MiraLAX)

Polyethylene Glycol 3350 is an osmotic laxative is used to soften stools and relieve constipation. Stress dietary changes that happen when disaster strikes often result in stomach and bowel problems.

Glycerin Suppositories

Constipation can be relieved in minutes with glycerin suppositories. They're a good backup to have if the polyethylene doesn't work.

Pseudoephedrine (Sudafed)

Pseudoephedrine is a decongestant that works well for

temporarily relieving the congestion of the upper and lower respiratory tract. It works well for treating the common cold, flu, hay fever, allergies, and bronchitis.

Pseudoephedrine-containing products are only available in pharmacies. You need to present an ID to obtain them. This is because it's used in manufacturing methamphetamine. You'll need to stock up on this medication over time.

Fexofenadine Hydrochloride (Allegra)

Fexofenadine is an antihistamine commonly used to relieve allergy symptoms. It's often taken along with pseudoephedrine to relieve allergy symptoms.

Meclizine (Bonine, Dramamine)

Drugs like this are used to treat nausea. Treatment eases nausea, vomiting, motion sickness, and vertigo-like dizziness. For some people, it helps relieve anxiety and insomnia.

Famotidine (Pepcid)

In late 2019, Zantac (ranitidine) was found to contain

high levels of NDMA. Because NDMA is associated with some cancers, all Zantac was pulled from the shelves.

Despite the low risk, doctors started using Pepcid (famotidine) instead of Zantac (ranitidine). It treats heartburn, ulcers, reflux and may help relieve hives.

Hydrocortisone Cream 1%

This cream is great for treating inflamed and/or itchy rashes.

Bacitracin Ointment (Baciguent)

This ointment treats abrasions, lacerations, insect bites, or stings. It doesn't work on fungus or virus infections. It can also treat superficial bacterial skin infections such as a mildly infected wound or impetigo.

Clotrimazole (Gyne-Lotrimin)

Clotrimazole is a topical antifungal medication. It can be used on fungal and yeast infections like the ones that cause yeast infections in women, athlete's foot, jock itch, ringworm, diaper rash and skinfold irritation.

Antacids

One of the most common conditions that people suffer from is acid reflux. This can be caused by many factors ranging from consuming highly acidic foods to chronic conditions such as stomach ulcers. Acid reflux is likely to happen at any time. You should always have anti-acid drugs in your house even if you are not preparing for the worst-case scenario.

The good news is that you can purchase as many antacids as you want from your local pharmacy without a prescription. The top three antacids that most people use are Pepcid, Nexium, and Zantac.

With most people having access to these drugs, you can purchase as much as you need in preparation for the worst-case scenario. Most antacids are simply Calcium Carbonate. In most situations where you cannot access antacids, you may want to turn to natural sources of calcium carbonate. These include morning cereals such as oatmeal. Other foods such as ginger, lean meats, and vegetables are also antacids.

In case you suffer from acid problems and lack access to the necessary medication, avoid highly acidic foods that may spike your stomach acid levels. The most common causes of high acidity include citrus fruits and some grains such as beans.

Cold and Flu Medicines

Flu and colds are common, especially during the cold season. Most people use flu shots to prevent the occurrence of the same. The problem in an SHFT event is that you won't have access to flu shots. If you want to be safe even in such an event, it is better to get your stock of flu shots now. Even if you do not have access to flu shots, you may still collect enough medicine to treat flu and colds.

The most commonly used flu medications you should stock up are analgesics such as acetaminophen (Tylenol) and Ibuprofen (Motrin). You may also use naproxen sodium (Aleve) which works effectively against common types of pain associated with colds.

With that in mind, flu and colds do not necessarily need medication to be treated. Your immune system is strong enough to fight off most flu attacks successfully. As long as you are leading a healthy lifestyle, most flu and cold attacks should go away in less than a week.

If you find the flu unbearable, you may use regular pain killers to make the situation better. You also have the choice of using herbal remedies to deal with flu and cold symptoms. Honey and lemon mixture works wonders in alleviating symptoms such as sore throats. The other remedies you may use include Chinese tea, thyme, and a ginger hot brew. These herbs are effective in loosening congestion caused by the flu.

Stockpiling Antibiotics for Disaster Preparedness

The other medical supplies you should stock up in preparation for the SHFT event are antibiotics. Virtually everyone on this earth has interacted with antibiotics in some way. Antibiotics are among the most popular and the most important medications on earth today due to the vital role they play in treating infections.

While antibiotics are important, they are not the bulletproof solution to every medical condition. I have seen people use antibiotics to treat diseases that cannot respond to such. You should know what antibiotics treat, the classes of antibiotics and how they are administered.

Antibiotics specifically treat infections caused by bacteria. The common bacteria that cause dangerous diseases include Staph, Strep. and E. coli. These are just but a few of the bacteria that are dangerous and can be treated by antibiotics.

You should think carefully about deciding to store antibiotics. Legally, antibiotics can only be prescribed by a doctor licensed to use the drug. They won't do anything to help a viral infection, but they can save lives.

Don't use antibiotics except under the direction of a qualified healthcare provider. The antibiotics you stockpile should only be used when competent medical care isn't available, and you don't have other safe options available to you.

In order to treat the condition, the correct antibiotic must be administered. It is important to carefully weigh the side effects of antibiotics before taking them. The best place to obtain antibiotics is from your healthcare provider.

According to Cynthia Koelker, the best antibiotics to store for emergency preparedness are Cephalexin, Ciprofloxacin, and Metronidazole. These three antibiotics cover 90% of common bacterial infections.

Cephalexin (Keflex)

This antibiotic treats most of the same bacteria amoxicillin does, but it's stronger against Staph aureus. The drug is commonly used to treat upper respiratory infections, skin infections, ear infections, and urinary tract infections.

Ciprofloxacin (Cipro)

This antibiotic is also used to treat bacterial infections. It could treat anthrax, typhoid fever, gastrointestinal infections, urinary tract infections, prostate infections, bone infections, pneumonia, and bronchitis.

Metronidazole (Flagyl)

Metronidazole treats parasitic infections like Giardia in the small intestine, amebic dysentery, and amebic liver abscesses. Infections of the stomach, liver, brain, respiratory tract, and vaginal canal can also be treated with it.

It is important to remember that antibiotics will not

work on viral infections. Viral infections are caused by viruses that cannot be inhibited by antibiotics. This is one reason why you are not allowed to use antibiotics to treat COVID-19. To help you understand the difference between antibiotics and other drugs. Let's look at disease-causing pathogens and their classification to understand more about antibiotics.

Disease-Causing Pathogens and Their Classification

There are four main types of pathogens that generally cause all of the diseases that affect the human body. Each of these classes of pathogens is treated with specific classes of medication. Although antibiotics are commonly used, they cannot fight all the pathogens that attack the human body.

The main disease-causing pathogens are classified into

Viruses

Bacteria

Fungi

Viruses

Viruses refer to protein layers that may take activity in the human body. Viruses are not living things, but they can significantly harm the human body. Viruses multiply very fast than any other disease-causing pathogen. They are also transferred quite faster. Traditionally, viruses have proven quite difficult to treat as compared to other pathogens. This is because they can easily shift shape.

Virus-caused diseases are treated using antiviruses. We will look at the best antivirus you can stock up in your prepper's pantry. With that said, most common viral infections rarely need treatment. These include flue, common colds, and others. More severe viral infections such as COVID-19 are best dealt with by getting the vaccine. While others, such as HIV, can only be managed given that there are no known medications for the virus.

Bacterial Infections

Bacterial infections are best treated using antibiotics. These are conditions caused by bacteria, as mentioned. With that in mind, not all types of bacterial infections are treated with the same type of antibiotics. The antibiotics you will use to treat whooping cough is not the same antibiotic used for UTIs. Although they are both bacterial infections, they are treated with different classes of antibiotics. I will show you the classes of antibiotics later on.

Fungus Infections

Fungus infections are caused by fungi. These conditions are commonly external but may also occur internally. A condition such as Athlete's foot is caused by a fungal attack on your feet. Internally, the most common fungus infections are oral thrush and virginal yeast. Oral thrush is a condition that may lead to bad breath and sores in the mouth. This and other fungus infections can only be treated with antifungal medication.

Parasite Infections

Parasite infections are caused by parasites. Tapeworms are probably the most common parasites that are known to cause tapeworm infection. Such conditions may affect an individual both internally and externally. When preparing your drugs, make sure to pack some antiparasitic drugs as well.

Conditions Commonly Treated with Antibiotics

As we have seen, antibiotics are very common and are used almost everywhere in the world. Unfortunately, if antibiotics are misused, they can cause severe problems. Among the dangers of antibiotic misuse include drug resistance and even severe symptoms. If you keep on using antibiotics to treat all conditions, your body may become resistant to antibiotics. This may mean that it will not respond to the drugs when you will need them

It is, therefore, necessary to know which antibiotics are used for which specific conditions. There are conditions that use light antibiotics and those that need strong antibiotics. The most common conditions that are treated with antibiotics include:

Acne	conjunctivitis (Pink Eye)	bronchitis
otitis media (ear infection)	sexually transmitted diseases (STDs)	Streptococcal Pharyngitis (Strep Throat)

Skin or Soft Tissue Infection	Upper respiratory tract infection	traveler's diarrhea

As you can see from my list, most of the common conditions that affect people around us are bacterial infections. This is a reason why antibiotics are very popular and commonly available in most homes.

Common Antibiotics

Although there are many antibiotics available in the market, there are those that are commonly available. These are antibiotics you can purchase over the counter without necessarily being required to provide a prescription. Because they are common and easily available, it is advisable to have each one of them in your medical stockpile. They include amoxicillin, doxycycline, cephalexin, ciprofloxacin, clindamycin, metronidazole, azithromycin, sulfamethoxazole, trimethoprim, and levofloxacin.

Classes of Antibiotics

Antibiotics come in different classes. There are so many classes of antibiotics we can't even mention them all. The classification of antibiotics is based on their strength, uses, and other factors such as the mode of manufacture, etc. When stockpiling antibiotics for your dark day, keep in mind that not all antibiotics are the same. There are those that are more effective against specific infections. There are also antibiotics that are more dangerous than others.

Below are some of the most common classes of antibiotics that you must consider when stocking up your drugs for doomsday.

Penicillin

This is one of the most common classes of antibiotics. It mainly contains five groups of antibiotics, namely aminopenicillin, beta-lactamase inhibitors, antipseudomonal penicillin, natural penicillin, penicillinase-resistant penicillin. These are mainly light antibiotics that are effective in treating common infections that do not cause severe symptoms.

Tetracyclines

These are broad-spectrum antibiotics that are normally administered to deal with diverse types of bacterial infections. They are used to treat conditions such as urinary tract infections, intestinal tract infections, STDs, and eye infections, among others. These common conditions are easily treated by broad-spectrum antibiotics. Examples of antibiotics in this category are demeclocycline, doxycycline, eravacycline.

Cephalosporins

There are currently up to 5 generations of cephalosporins. These are antibiotics that are tailored to counter changes in different bacterial infections. They are mainly key in treating gram-negative infections. Examples of these antibiotics are cefaclor, a second-generation antibiotic and cefadroxil, the first-generation drug.

Quinolones

The other class of antibiotics that you want to purchase is quinolones. This class is mainly made up of synthetic antibacterial drugs with broad-spectrum activity. Most of the antibiotics in this class have a broad spectrum application but are classified under quinolones due to the fact that they are synthetic.

With these drugs being mainly synthetic, they have more side effects than other antibiotics. As a result, the FDA discourages the use of quinolones for infections that can be treated by other classes of antibiotics. With that said, most quinolones are quite strong and can effectively deal with infections that can not be treated with other antibiotics. Examples of antibiotics that fall within this group are moxifloxacin and ciprofloxacin.

Lincomycin

The other class of antibiotics you should consider purchasing for the SHFT event is lincomycin. This class of antibiotics is hailed for its effectiveness against gram-positive aerobes and anaerobes. It can also work against some gram-negative anaerobe. This type of antibiotic is used to treat serious infections such as pelvic inflammatory disease, lower respiratory tract infections, and abdominal infections, among others.

Generally, there are over ten classes of antibiotics which are further broken down into sub-classes. When stocking up antibiotics for the SHFT event, make sure to get a piece of the different classes. As you can see from above, each of the classes has its uses and purposes. Therefore, it is important you purchase drugs that are diverse in nature.

The other classes of antibiotics you may want to consider when making bulk purchases include:

Macrolides

Sulfonamides

Glycopeptides

Aminoglycosides

Carbapenems

Each of these classes its pros and cons. Consider getting the right information from the vendor before purchasing. You may want to inquire about factors such as side effects, expiration dates, age groups that can use the drugs, among other information.

Do not just go around administering all types of

antibiotics to everybody. For instance, quinolones are not supposed to be administered to children under any circumstance. If you end up stocking up on these antibiotics alone, you might find yourself in more trouble when you need help.

Specialized Drugs for Specific Risks

Depending on your specific risk factors, there may be unique situations you're preparing for that require special drugs to be used.

Potassium Iodide (KI)

This is taken during a nuclear disaster to prevent the thyroid gland from absorbing radiation. If you're preparing to survive nuclear war, this is a must-have. As long as you store it in a cool, dry, dark location in its original container, it should remain stable for many years.

Oseltamivir (Tamiflu)

This antiviral medication requires a prescription. It's used to treat or prevent influenza. You may want to consider purchasing it if you're prepping for a pandemic.

Zanamivir (Relenza)

Zanamivir is an antiviral powder that's inhaled orally. Zanamivir is used to both treat and prevent the flu and requires a prescription to purchase.

Bee Sting Remedies

In a situation where you can't access medical care, you have to factor in how to deal with many unique situations. One of those unique situations is bee stings. When you are stung by a bee or a wasp, you should have an immediate solution to alleviate the pain. Multiple bee stings can be poisonous and even lead to death if not taken care of.

Any person stung by bees should use antihistamines such as diphenhydramine (Benadryl) and nose dilating drugs such as loratadine (Claritin). These drugs can help with itchiness and are effective in reducing the swelling caused by bee stings. You should also use acetaminophen (Tylenol) or ibuprofen (Motrin) for pain relief.

Snake Bite Remedies

You are more likely to be bitten by a snake in SHFT

situations. At such a time, people may be disconnected from power, and modern living styles may be completely out of reach. You may even be operating in the jungle, where you encounter snakes on a daily basis. This calls for preparedness against snake bites since most poisonous snakes can kill a person within minutes.

The ideal drugs to stock for snake bites are anti venomous drugs. Ideally, you should have a few doses of antivenom (Crotalidae) polyvalent systemic drug class. You may also want to stock some antitoxins with some pain relief medicine.

In case of a snake bite, caution should be taken first. Antivenom medicine should be administered immediately in the required dosages. In case the victim is long-distance from the drug, first aim measures should be taken. To prevent the venom from traveling to the rest of the body, techniques such as tightening a bandage on both sides of the bite are recommended.

In some situations, an experienced individual may suck out the venom and spit it to the ground. Do not attempt these techniques unless you have no other way out. Sucking the venom can be dangerous, especially for individuals who have never had such an experience before.

Wilderness Medicine vs. Long-Term Survival Medicine

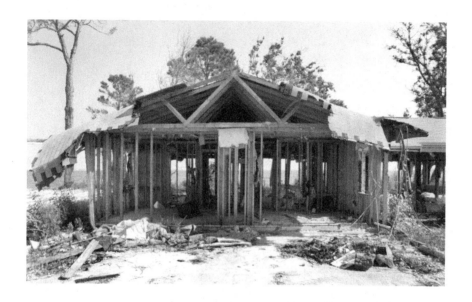

Wilderness Medicine

What's the difference between wilderness medicine and long-term survival medicine? Wilderness medicine is defined as medical care given in a situation where modern care, training, and facilities aren't available. It's usually given during wilderness hikes, maritime expeditions, and journeys into developing countries.

There are trained doctors and modern hospitals, but they aren't available at the time that medical care is required - maybe for a significant period of time. Since you're the temporary caregiver, you'll be responsible for stabilizing the patient. That means you can't allow the illness or injury to get worse.

Your primary goal will be to evacuate the patient to a modern medical facility, even if it is hundreds of miles away from the patient's location. Once you've transferred the patient to the next highest medical resource, your responsibility to the sick or injured person will be over. Emergency medical technicians or military corpsmen will recognize the strategy as "stabilize and transport."

Long-Term Survival Medicine

Non-physicians can benefit from wilderness classes, EMT training, and even military medical corps training. It is extremely helpful to have this training if you have the time. A short-term deficit of medical assistance is more likely than a long-term one.

Despite this, you'll have to plan for the possibility that you may be completely alone one day. The way you think about this must change to fit a day when intensive care units and emergency rooms are inaccessible. You won't be able to pass the sick or injured person along to a formally trained provider, so you must be prepared to remain with your patient throughout the entire process.

Therefore, you need to learn methods that will work in a power-down situation. It is even possible to turn to older strategies that modern medicine might consider obsolete. If you use a combination of prevention, improvisation, and prudent use of supplies, you should be able to handle most problems a power outage causes.

Enlist the help of others.

When you're trying to stockpile emergency medicine for a disaster, it's important that you enlist the help of others. Community is important because if you try to go it alone, you'll most likely end up extinct, like the Tasmanian wolf.

There's no better time than now to communicate, network, and put together a group of like-minded people. The right number of able people for a mutual assistance group depends on your retreat and your resources. The ideal group has people with diverse skills but similar philosophies.

Unless you're already in a community like this, you may feel like it's not possible to form a support system. That's not the case - you'll find many people in online forums about preparedness.

It's not enough just to be in a group, though. The people in that group need to meet regularly, decide on priorities and set things in motion. Put together plans A, B, and C and work together to implement them successfully. Keep the lines of communication open so that your group members are kept informed.

Take care of your health before a catastrophe happens.

If you, as a medical caregiver, don't set an example of good health and fitness, how do you expect anyone else to? You can accomplish this by:

Maintaining a normal weight based on your height and age.

Eating a healthy diet.

Maintaining good hygiene.

Staying physically fit.

Eliminating unhealthy habits like smoking and others.

Managing current medical issues quickly.

It's important to tune up any chronic medical problems you might have. For instance, make sure your blood pressure is under control. If you have a badly broken knee, you might want to get it fixed surgically so that you can function well when the going gets tough. Use modern technology while you have it.

You should also deal with dental problems before modern times make dentistry unavailable.

If you have bad habits, work to eliminate them. If you damage your heart and lungs with smoking, how will you function in a situation requiring fitness and stamina? If you drink alcohol a lot or use drugs, how do you expect anyone to trust your judgment in critical situations?

Paying careful attention to hygiene is also important for your success in times of trouble. Those who don't maintain sanitary conditions in their retreat will have a difficult time staying healthy. In a collapse, infections that are usually seen only in underdeveloped countries, such as different types of viruses and bacteria, will become commonplace, and essential medical supplies will include things like soap and bleach.

These two basic strategies will take you a long way in your journey to being prepared for a collapse. They don't cost anything and will give you the best chance of success if everything else fails.

How to Stockpile Supplies Without Looking Crazy

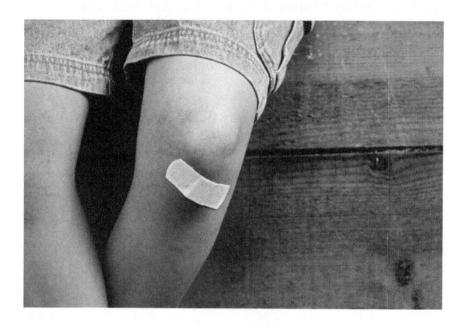

When you decide to start stockpiling supplies, others may look at you like you're crazy. There are ways to stockpile supplies without looking crazy, though. We'll cover them here.

Set a Goal

Decide how much you wish to store. Do you need How about three months? You should stock up on emergency supplies based on the kind of emergency that is likely to occur where you live and how long you anticipate being without supplies.

According to the federal government, you should have at least a three-day supply of food and water for each member of your household

The list of supplies also includes a flashlight, battery-powered or hand-cranked radio, and basic first-aid supplies.

If you want an all-in-one solution, the American Red Cross offers 3-Day emergency preparedness kits and other emergency supplies. You can also check Amazon for emergency and survival kits

In a crisis, you can feel much safer if you go more than 72 hours beyond the bare minimum. When you reach that goal, move it to one or two weeks. Maintain this for as long as you need to.

Face the Challenges

Stockpiling medical supplies can be one of the most challenging situations. You might even find yourself being tracked by law enforcement unless you go about it the right way. Keep in mind that what you are doing at this point may not be legal. You may not be allowed to buy medical supplies for no intended use and stock them in your house. Given that we are preparing for a situation that might mean life or death, this is a decision you have to make. You have to decide to do that which the law prohibits. After all, especially in an SHFT scenario, no one operates under the law.

Piling up medical supplies may make you look crazy, even to your own family members. Even before you start taking this step, you should make sure that your family members understand what you are doing. In case you have children who are too young to understand what you are doing, keep them out of the conversation.

Secondly, you will most definitely look crazy if people find out you are pilling up medical supplies for the unknown. Therefore, it is a good idea to keep your operations as secretive as possible. One of the few ways of not being seen as a mad man is by keeping your operations secretive.

Storing Water

Water should be prioritized and stored safely.

For each person, the CDC recommends storing one gallon of water per day and establishing a two-week supply if possible. If you have pets, you should also store extra water. According to the CDC, unopened, commercially bottled water is the safest and most reliable emergency water supply.

If you want to, you can also store tap water in your own containers.

The CDC provides these tips for storing water:

1. If you use store-bought water, check the expiration dates and replace it as needed.

2. Replace the water you have stored yourself every six months.

3. Keep unscented liquid chlorine bleach in your emergency supplies for cleaning and sanitizing.

4. If the bleach contains cleaning additives or color-safe

dye, do not use it. The product should be labeled as safe for water disinfection.

Buy Bulk Supplies

To stockpile affordably, especially if you have a large household or want a full, long-lasting stockpile, purchase in bulk.

To save money if you do not belong to a warehouse club, check out what foods your local Walmart sells in economy size, such as a four-pound jar of peanut butter for $4 - or check out many foods that Amazon sells in bulk sizes.

Ways to Be Secretive with Your Stash

To achieve secrecy, there are specific things you should do. These include:

Limit Access to the Drug Store Room

Before you start ordering supplies, make sure you have a room dedicated to drug storage. This room should be set apart with limited access. Limiting access to the storeroom is helpful in many ways. For instance, since the room has drugs, limiting access helps protect children who may end up misusing the drugs. Secondly, it helps hide your secret of gathering drugs from neighbors and other visitors who may be interested in knowing what you are up to.

Shred Receipts and other Proof of Shopping Documents

One of the things that will make people know that you are stocking medicine is when you throw your receipts in the bin. The receipts may find their way in the wrong hands, and people will start questioning why you purchase huge amounts of medical supplies.

Transport all Supplies in Your Personal Car

Even though online shopping is an option, I highly recommend shopping in places where you can collect the supplies yourself. If you drive into your parking with a box of drugs, a few people may suspect what you are doing. However, if a medical supplies van keeps on parking at your gate, people will start becoming suspicious.

How to Obtain Bulk Medical Supplies

There are tricks you may use to get access to bulk supplies of medicine and other medical necessities without raising concern. You do not even want your closest neighbor to know about your operations. For this reason, try concealing your workings as much as possible. Among the ways you can use to stock up supplied include:

Link Up With Local Pharmacists to Order Supplies

You may be unable to order bulk drugs from the supply agencies yourself, but you will find it easy if you use local pharmacists. If you have a good relationship with a local pharmacist, you may request their assistance in getting certain medications and tools. The good news is that such a person might also be helpful in providing guidance on how the drugs are used.

Register as a Pharmacy, Hire a Pharmacist and Obtain a License

The other option would be registering a pharmacist. The steps involved in the registration of pharmacists can be quite complex but are achievable. If you fail to find any other way of obtaining bulk drugs and other supplies, you may want to register a pharmacist. This will mean you will either have to obtain pharmacy training or work with someone who is a trained pharmacist.

What most people do is that, although they may lack qualifications to run a pharmacy, they enter into a partnership with a qualified pharmacist. The pharmacist acts as a partner in the business, which in turn gives the other partner access to the medical supplies provided.

Register a Limited Liability Company (LLC)

One of the major ways that people protect their wealth is by registering limited companies. If you have a home where you live and would like to store up medical supplies for the future, you could register your home as a base for a private company. However, you have to specify what your company does, how many employees you have, where you are located, along with other factors.

The beauty of registering your home as a private company is that you will not be directly liable for every action you take. Secondly, companies and institutions such as schools are allowed to order over-the-counter medications in bulk. You must be aware that most schools have nurses or even clinics. These clinics are part of the institution. When a school orders bulk medical supplies, fewer questions will be asked as compared to a situation where an individual orders bulk medical supplies.

Shop Gradually and Smart

The best and easiest way to stock up medication without getting suspected by anyone is to go about it in a systematic manner. The laws are clear on how to obtain medication from a hospital or from a pharmacist. In most cases, you will need a medical prescription.

If you suffer from a specific condition that may need long-term supplies, you can easily get a prescription for it. Once you have your written prescription, visit a pharmacist and purchase your drugs. You can still use the same prescription in a hundred other pharmacists and collect the drugs. In one day, you can collect as many drugs to serve you for the whole year.

The other alternative is to use the emergency script. This is a bit risky but works most of the time. Let's say you want to stock up supplies for conditions such as asthma. Even if you do not have a prescription, you can simply show up at a local pharmacist and pretend to be in an emergency. Although most pharmacists need a prescription, they will easily sell you the drugs if you are in an emergency situation without asking more questions.

Foods to Stockpile for Emergency Use

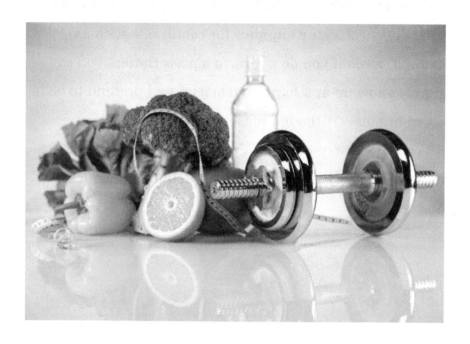

Eating from a stockpile can get boring. The following list has foods that not only need no cooking and are nutritionally dense but also are tasty. They include:

Peanut butter

Whole wheat crackers (vacuum pack these to prolong freshness)

Nuts and trail mix.

Cereal - buy these in individual packaging to prolong their freshness.

Power bars and granola bars.

Dried fruits.

Canned tuna, salmon, chicken, and turkey

Canned vegetables such as beans, carrots, and peas.

Canned soups and chili.

Sports drinks - avoid those that have sugar and artificial color.

Sugar, salt, and pepper.

Powdered milk.

In addition, there are 11 foods that will keep for years. They are:

Oats

White rice

Popcorn

Dark chocolate

Honey

Powdered milk.

Dried beans.

Certain cheeses - according to Dairy Foods
Magazine, low moisture hard cheeses such as
parmesan and aged cheddar can last from 10 months to
several years.

Commercially canned foods - when buying canned
foods, avoid cans that are rusted, dented, scratched or
bulging.

Frozen foods.

Sugar

Don't forget a can opener!

Seeds

Include seeds to sprout. You should keep some vegetable, nut, and grain seeds on hand for sprouting.

Beans - They're easy to grow and preserve. They're high in fiber, calcium, and vitamins A, C, and K.

Spinach - This vegetable does well in cold weather, and it's prolific. Many people call it a superfood because it has many different vitamins like Vitamin A, C, iron, thiamine, and folic acid.

Carrots - This crop does well in cold weather and requires very little space to grow. It's high in carbohydrates, vitamin A, and vitamin C.

Squash and pumpkin are both prolific producers. Both store well, especially winter squash. You can save the seeds or roast them and eat them. There are lots of carbohydrates in squash, as well as Vitamins A and C, magnesium, and potassium.

Allium varieties - These include onions, shallots, leeks, and garlic. They contain fiber, Vitamin B6, Vitamin C, folate, and potassium.

Beets - They're easy to grow and multi-functional. You can consume both the roots and greens, which make beets a dual-purpose crop.

When pest issues are kept to a minimum, tomatoes can produce a lot of food from a small space. Tomatoes contain Vitamins A, C, K, E, potassium, thiamine, and niacin.

Broccoli - This is another cool-weather vegetable. It contains a lot of protein, vitamins A and K, and carbohydrates.

Peppers - Peppers such as cayenne are essential for natural remedies. Each variety is rich in vitamins A and C.

Eggplant - Most people wouldn't think to grow this vegetable, but it's still a good one. It's relatively easy to grow and can grow for three or more years. Plus, it's pretty easy to save seeds from.

Asparagus - This one is an essential perennial. Depending on the region, established asparagus plants can continue to produce for 30 years - some report for longer.

Amaranth - This is another dual-purpose plant. It's naturally drought tolerant. You can use the seeds of this plant as a grain - just cook it the same way you would cook Quinoa. The leaves can be picked while they're young and tender and eaten raw or sauteed the same way you would cook spinach.

Radish - if you want a crop that matures fast, radishes are one of the best. Radishes are mature in as few as 25 days from seeds to harvest. The seeds are easy to save from crops and just as easy to stockpile.

Corn - This one deserves a specific mention. Corn isn't the easiest crop to grow, but it has many uses. Most people think of sweet corn. However, dent corn and field corn are also important. Both can be dried to feed livestock. You can also dry it and make it into cornmeal.

Other Foods to Include

Herbs - Natural pest control can be obtained through companion planting with herbs. Medicinal herbs are important for making herbal remedies.

Flowers - Flowers can be used for companion planting

and to attract bees for pollination. The best flowers to use are borage, purple cornflower, marigolds, nasturtium, plains coreopsis, cornflower, yarrow, sunflowers, and calendula.

Potatoes - Remember, seed potatoes do not keep. You need to continually replenish your stock from your own crops. Potatoes are a staple in many people's diets, especially those in the west. They contain potassium, copper and B6 and are really good to fill you up at mealtime. They are usually pretty easy to grow, although some varieties are very disease-prone.

When possible, stock up on longer-lasting fresh items.

If you see trouble coming and can buy fresh foods, Real Simple recommends items that can ask for weeks or months if stored properly. These include:

Apples

Citrus fruit.

Winter squashes such as acorn squash.

Potatoes and yams.

Rotate Food Rations

Check the shelf life of your stored food regularly to make sure it's safe and nutritious when you need it. Make use of foods nearing the end of their shelf life by rotating them in the kitchen. You can then add fresh supplies to the stockpile.

Handling Medical Situations

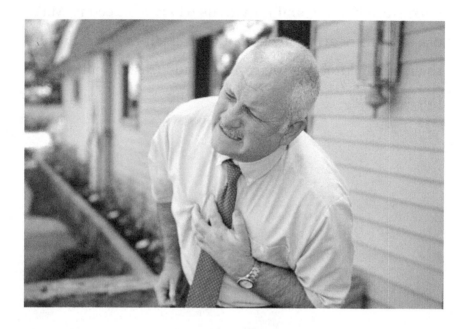

If you have to deal with a medical situation in a crisis, it's important to know how to respond in that situation. The following steps will help you gain knowledge of the situation and respond appropriately.

As soon as possible, provide a sense of hope, safety, and connectedness, regardless of whether the person is conscious or unconscious - In a high-stress, dangerous situation, most information is processed subconsciously. It is possible for the unconscious to remember sounds, smells, and sights.

Try to remain calm, look the person in the eye, and avoid expressing. Our non-verbal cues often contradict our words, so stay in control and aware of your body language.

Remove blood, mud, and debris from the person's face. Calm the environment. Consider covering them with a blanket, removing bystanders, and reducing the lights or sirens if possible. These are the things that can cause anxiety and feelings of distress and fear.

Demonstrate care and listen to others. Showing you care will make you more trustworthy. If you want someone to listen to you or act on your advice, you need to gain their trust. Listening, caring, empathy, and compassion are crucial to trust-building. Within the first 9 to 30 seconds of an interaction, people decide how much trust to place in you, so you need to make a good first impression. Gain trust and show that you care by paraphrasing what people say, validating their feelings, and reassuring them.

Show competence and expertise as well as honesty and openness. Talk to the person throughout the caregiving process. If you explain what you are doing and what they can expect when providing treatment or aid, it can help calm people. By giving the person tasks, they can feel in charge. Be honest about what you know and don't know. If you tell the truth, they are more likely to follow your directions. Don't over-reassure the person with statements you can't back up.

Communicate clearly and concisely, using short messages and repeating as necessary. During stressful situations, people tend to concentrate on what they hear first. In a crisis, a person's ability to process information can be reduced by up to 80%. You may have to repeat important facts in the event of a crisis since people may find it difficult to hear, understand, and remember.

Use positive language, such as "you will survive." Avoid negatives, such as "you won't die." Mental processing is primarily visual. A person's subconscious mind focuses on the negative rather than the positive throughout this example, even focusing on the word "die." People often focus on the negative rather than the positive. Studies show that people have a hard time understanding negative statements

Communicate indirectly if direct communication is met with resistance. Say, for example, "I don't know when you will feel better," where the command comes after an unassuming set-up phrase. Use this kind of setup before delivering a command that is delivered in a different tempo, volume, or intensity to encourage the person to respond positively.

Recognize that people may perceive risk as high. People tend to magnify sights, smells, sounds, and feelings in high-stress situations. They see things differently and think they're at risk. Messages or information that are perceived as high-risk can be processed differently. Do not get frustrated if they don't understand you right away. You should continue to reassure people, so they understand your direction. Don't be frustrated if you aren't understood right away.

Handling Mass Casualties

If you find yourself in a position where you have to provide medical care to many people, you must be well prepared for the situation. In a pandemic or war situation, doctors easily get overwhelmed by patients. You should have a clear plan on how to handle the available patients. You should decide which patients are given priority and how the other patients should be handled. Although we are preparing for a time when medical practices may not be useful, you may want to use some of the principles applied by doctors in handling patients. Health professionals follow a procedure that leads to the lowest possible casualties in every situation. The principles to follow are:

The Most Critically Ill Patient Should Be Given Priority

Whenever an emergency case is brought into a hospital, doctors have to stop most of their other duties to attend to the emergency first. The critically ill patient should be given a chance to survive by being accorded the best treatment possible. Using this approach will help you know who to attend to first and who last. With that said, in an SHFT situation, all patients may be critical.

You should be able to use your judgment well. In this situation, you should remember that your hands are tied. You probably do not have the necessary tools to handle complex medical care procedures. Instead of wasting time on a critically ill patient who has zero chances of survival, it is better to channel your energy to a patient who may survive. As the medical care provider, you want to gauge the possibility of a person recovering. Do not just waste all your resources on a patient that has minimal chances of survival.

Open Wounds Should Be Given Priority

Once you have dealt with those who may die if not given attention, you want to turn to those who have openly exposed wounds. Do not start treating people who look okay when there are those with open wounds. The problem with having open wound patients is that bleeding may contaminate your working space. For a medical practitioner, you want your operating space to remain as clean as possible. Any person who may mess up with your room must be handled promptly. These include people with exposed wounds.

Give Priority to Special Groups

The other group of patients you want to look at well are those in special classes. For instance, pregnant women should be given priority in a long queue where all patients may not get attention. In war situations, women and children are given the first priority. In a situation such as the COVID-19 pandemic, the elderly were given priority. This is because they are a highly vulnerable group. Again remember that the way you triage and treat your patients will be at your own discretion. However, the best way out will include offering help to amateurs that guarantees safety for all the parties involved.

Isolate Highly Contagious Cases

The other key principle of triaging patients is isolation. When people come in for treatment, the first step should be asking for their symptoms. If a person has symptoms that may resemble those of a contagious disease, they should be isolated. Probably, you may not have all the equipment to carry out tests for all conditions.

However, by listening to your patients and comparing symptoms, you should be able to tell if someone could be a patient of some specific disease. Diseases outbreaks are common scenarios across the world.

For example, in the ace of Ebola in Africa, patients could be seen oozing out blood. These are obvious signs that caregivers can use to separate infected patients from uninfected ones.

Focus on Treatable Conditions

Although all patients should be given a chance to survive, do not spend too much time on conditions that cannot be treated. This is one principle that is not easy to handle. There are situations where you will have to see people dying. Just because there is no way you can help them, you will have to move on and save those that can be saved in an SHFT situation; the case gets worse. In such difficult times, people tend to be a bit more selfish. You should try to be considerate of all patients but remember that in all scenarios, there are casualties.

Save the Most Valuable Assets

In war or any kind of disaster, the medical practice principles require you to save the most valuable asset at the time. For instance, if two people pass out on a flying airplane- one being a pilot and the other passenger- you will be required to save the pilot first. Although the life of the passenger is equally important, if the pilot dies, the chances of the rest of the crew members dying are high. Saving the pilot will be the only way out if you want to save the entire crew.

This mostly applies in war situations. If there is war, soldiers and doctors may be given priority over civilians. They provide valuable services that will help the team continue fighting. An SHFT event means simply anything. It can be water, an earthquake, a disease outbreak, or anything else. You must keep all these scenarios in mind when preparing for the worst.

The way you triage patients and attend to them will determine their chances of getting well. If you are responsible for this type of organization, avoid a situation where the waiting bay causes more serious damages than the conditions at hand.

Use the SALT Method to Triage Patients

When a lot of people need medical care, you need to know how to triage these patients and decide who gets treated first. The following guide will provide some basic information on how to decide which patients get treated first

The SALT method applies in situations where you have five or more people who need care. The acronym stands for Sort, Assess, Lifesaving Interventions, Treatment/Transport.

Sort

The first thing you'll do is sort patients according to the severity of their injuries. You could use the following categories:

Green (minimal treatment needed)

Yellow (Treatment can be delayed)

Red (Immediate treatment needed)

Black (dead)

You could also include an additional category, Gray, which means the patient is expected to die. If the patient is still breathing but is obviously badly injured, they wouldn't need immediate treatment if they were obviously going to die soon.

Assess and Lifesaving Interventions

These two go hand in hand. For example, if you see a

patient's airway is obstructed, open it.

However, you should perform a lifesaving intervention only if it doesn't take too long. Opening a person's airway may not take very long, but If the lifesaving intervention you need to do requires getting the equipment you don't have access to, you might have to consider doing something else.

Treatment/Transport

Once you've assessed them and performed lifesaving interventions on those that need them, it's time to treat and/or transport the rest. Give treatment to those that you determined treatment can be delayed on, and transport the ones that are dead to a place where you can bury them.

Basic First Aid and CPR procedures

Once you've sorted people into groups based on the severity of their injuries, how do you treat them? This section will outline some basic first aid and CPR procedures.

What is CPR?

CPR stands for cardiopulmonary resuscitation. It's a potentially life-saving procedure that can restart a person's heartbeat and breathing. Usually, it is used to revive those who have suffered electric shocks, near-drownings, and heart attacks. Quick CPR can triple a person's chance of survival, according to the National Institutes of Health.

When to Use CPR?

Before you perform CPR, check to see if the person is responding. Ask them if they're ok and touch them on the shoulder. If he responds or is breathing, you don't need to do CPR. If they don't respond, you need to get emergency help right away. If you're alone, you may need to leave them for a few moments to call for emergency help. The purpose of CPR is to keep a victim alive until help arrives. If you're alone, you may need to start CPR immediately rather than calling 911 first.

Before you call 911, perform CPR on an infant or child who is unresponsive for two minutes. Attempting to open an infant's airway immediately before calling 911 is a common cause of cardiac arrest in children.

If an adult is unresponsive and has been the victim of near-drowning, trauma or drug overdose, the American Heart Association says it's more important to start CPR immediately than delay while you call 911.

How to Perform CPR

Performing hands-only CPR

People without CPR training can use the following steps to perform hands-only CPR:

1. Check the scene - make sure it's safe for you to reach the person who needs help.

2. See if the person responds. Shake their shoulder and ask them loudly if they're ok. For an infant, tap the bottom of their foot and wait for a reaction.

3. If the person isn't responsive, get help immediately - call 911 or your local emergency services if the person doesn't respond. Another person can also call. You should begin CPR if you believe the person drowned, or if they're a child between 1 and 8 years old, then call 911.

4. Identify hand position - If you are dealing with an adult, place your heel between their nipples in the center of their chest. Your other hand should be on top. Make sure your fingers are drawn up, and your heel is on their chest. For children between 1-8 years old, use one of your hands in the center of their chest. If you're reviving an infant, place two fingers in the center of their chest, slightly below the nipple line.

5. Begin compressions. When performing compressions on an adult, use your upper body to push straight down on their chest for at least two inches. Press 100 to 120 times per minute. Let their chest rest between compressions. Push straight down about two inches on the chest of children between the ages of 1 and 8 at a speed of 100 to 120 compressions per minute. Let their chest recoil between compressions.

6. Continue compressions. Repeat the cycle until the person starts to breathe or medical help arrives. If the person starts breathing, have them lie on their side quietly until medical help arrives.

How to Deal with Other Common Emergencies

There are other unique situations that can occur in a doomsday kind of scenario. For instance, the war experienced in Ukraine is a reminder that things can go from good to worse in a matter of hours. It is, therefore, necessary to also prepare for emergencies that may arise as a result of such emergencies.

These emergencies include gunshot wounds, electrocution, radiation exposure, among others.

Gunshot Wounds

A gunshot wound in an SHFT situation can lead to death. Gunshots must be attended to immediately to increase the chances of survival. One of the ways to ensure that the victim does not die is by preventing the gun poison from spreading in the body.

The first step to take when a person is shot is to tie the gunshot wound with a bandage to prevent excessive blood flow. If you do not have a bandage, use a piece of clean cloth. You do not want to use a piece that will contaminate the wound and lead to more infections. After tightening the wound, find a safe place to operate on the wound.

The best solution to gunshot wounds is removing the bullet. In an SHFT situation, you are not expecting to see a doctor soon, and hence you must gather the courage to take out the bullet yourself. Start by analyzing the state of the wound and its location. If the bullet is lodged in vital organs such as the heart or the brain, the best bet would be living it in there. However, if the bullet is lodged in the leg, arm, or less dangerous parts, you should move on and get it removed.

The first thing you will have to do is find a quiet place where the patient can lay flat on their back or tummy. This should provide ample working space. Find a piece of cloth, a pair of tweezers, or something similar that can be used to pull the bullet out. Let the patient relax before you start the operation.

To remove the bullet, you will need some form of a numbing application. If you have not stoked any medication that can be used for local anesthesia, try finding some. If you do not have any numbing medication, regular painkillers may help make the process less painful.

The next step is to tighten a piece of cloth around the bullet wound. This helps reduce the pain felt when the bullet is removed and also prevents excessive blood flow. If it is on areas such as the leg or thigh, tighten both sides of the bullet wound.

When the wound is well tightened, let the patient relax and start the operation. To relax the muscles around the bullet, pour surgical spirit into it. If you do not have spirit, you may use any form of alcohol. The spirit will jolt the bullet, making it come up slightly. Gently grab it with the tweezers and toggle it gently as you pull out. Although painful, keep on pulling gently until the bullet comes out.

Once you have the bullet out, expect a rush of blood out. Apply some spirit on a piece of cotton wool and use it to wash the wound. Once the wound is clean, bandage it with a clean bandage and let it heal.

Electrocution

Electrocution accidents can lead to serious injuries. In

most cases, electrocution may lead to death. To prevent death, those who are around a person being electrocuted should cut off power. The only way to protect the victim is by switching off the source of power. If it is not possible to turn off the source of power, the other option would be moving the victim away from the power source. For instance, in case a power supply line snaps and electrocutes someone, the only help that can be provided is moving the victim from the line.

To move a patient from the power source, use a dry non-conducting object such as wood. Using a conductor may get you electrocuted as well. If you touch the victim with your bare hands, you may also get electrocuted.

When a person is electrocuted, they may suffer various injuries. These include skin burns, interrupting blood flow, and even a heart attack. To help the patient, some steps should be taken as soon as the power has been cut off. There are many steps you can take as the primary caregiver. Among the steps you should take are:

Give the patient mouth to mouth CPR to assist the heart continue pumping blood. This is especially when you do not feel a pulse or when there are no signs of blood circulation.

If the patient has any burns, apply a bandage. Target the burned areas, covering them with a sterile gauze bandage. Make sure you purchase sufficient sterile gauze bandages in your stock. You will need them more than you will need other medical supplies in an SHFT scenario.

If you do not have a bandage when electrocution happens, you may also use a piece of clean cloth. You want to pick a very clean cotton cloth. Do not use a towel or blanket to avoid a situation where the fibers get stuck on the wounds.

With that, your patient should be stable and ready for further treatment. When the patient regains stability, you may want to use your medical supplies to enhance healing. If you have stocked any anti-burn creams, this is the time to apply them according to instructions. A person who has undergone electrocution must also undergo stabilization in terms of heart functions. Closely monitor the patient, listening to their heartbeat to determine if the heart is functioning properly. If a patient undergoes a heart attack, you may want to implement some of the steps we have discussed on heart attacks.

Radiation Exposure

In the event a person is exposed to radiation, all the other parties must be careful about how the situation is handled. Radioactive accidents can occur in the lab or in industries. Besides these places, in a war scenario, nuclear weapons may be used, releasing radiation. Being exposed to radiation can cause serious damage to the health of the victim. Both internal and external contamination of the body with radiation can be avoided based on the steps taken.

Acute exposure to radiation may lead to burns on the skin. It can also damage the brain, interfere with blood circulation and mess up the digestion system. Worse yet, the effects of radiation exposure may stay with a person for life.

In case a person is exposed to radiation, these are the steps you should take to help them survive the situation.

Ask the patient to move away from the exposure. The first aid attendants must always keep a distance of at least 100 meters from the source of the radiation. If there is a fire or an explosion that has been caused by the radioactive source, you should not be exposed to the fire or smoke from such an incidence.

If the source of exposure is sealed, there should be no problem approaching the scene.

Ideally, you should avoid moving close to a contaminated person. However, in a case where you are in a position to help, make sure you wear protective gear. Ideally, you should cover your entire body with radioactive protective wear. This is a type of clothing that is specifically designed to offer protection against radiation.

In case you do not have radiation-safe clothing, consider covering yourself in thick clothing from top to bottom or cover yourself with a plastic bag or both. This may reduce your exposure to radiation when attending to the patient.

Once you get access to the patient, the first step should be to remove all the clothing they are wearing and discard them away from environments where people live.

If the patient has buns, cover them well with a bandage before applying anti-burn treatment.

Besides treating the burns, those who suffer from radioactive injuries may use painkillers to reduce the pain. You may also administer drugs that help control diarrhea and vomiting.

Generally, there are no drugs that can reverse the effects of radiation exposure. Most people who are severely exposed to radiation may die within two to three days. In situations where the exposure is not too serious, the patient may have to live with the pain associated with the burns for a long time. In some situations, permanent deformities may occur.

Your role as the primary medical person in an SHFT situation is to stabilize the patient. Provide medication that can give the patient some comfort. If any part of the body is severely hurt, you may even be forced to perform an amputation. At the end of the day, the care you provide should help the patient feel comfortable and get a chance to live again. This is one of the hardest situations to handle.

Heart Attack

A heart attack can occur when you are out of reach from medical assistance. In such a situation, you should be able to offer primary care in order to stabilize the patient. Similar to cardiac arrests, a heart attack can also cause a person to lose consciousness. However, it is rarer for an individual undergoing a heart attack to lose consciousness.

When a person is experiencing a heart attack, the first step you should take is CPR. Perform a mouth-to-mouth CPR if you do not feel a pulse or if the person is not breathing. The CPR helps blood to continue flowing through the body, giving the patient a higher chance of survival.

While performing CPR, push hard in the center of the chest with continuous pumping. Pump at approximately 100 to 120 compressions per minute. These actions should help the heart restore normal functioning before the patient passes away.

Once the heart attack has been stopped, give the patient some Aspirin. Aspirin may help keep the blood from clotting and reduce heart damage. Make sure your patient is not allergic to Aspirin before administering it to avoid complicating the situation.

Once your patient is in a stable condition, you may

want to go back to regular heart condition drugs mentioned above. Make sure you know which drugs can be taken to keep your patient stable for a while.

Medical Terms Everyone Should Know

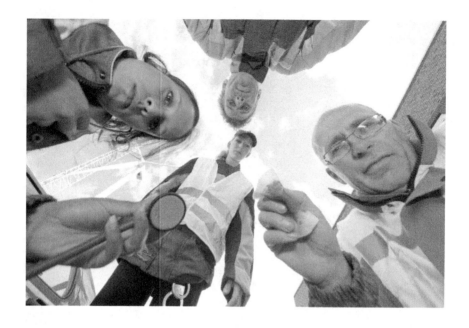

This book contains plenty of new terms you may not be familiar with. Here are some of the terms that you may want to learn about in regards to medical care. In an emergency situation, there are certain terms everyone should know. This section will provide definitions of those medical terms.

Abrasion - A cut or scrape that typically isn't serious. These are usually handled at levels of primary health care.

Abscess - A tender, fluid-filled pocket that forms in tissue, usually because of infection.

Acute - Describes a condition that begins abruptly and is sometimes severe, but the duration of the condition is short. Most such conditions are likely to cause death.

Benign: Something that does not cause cancer.

Biopsy: Refers to a small tissue sample that is collected from the patient to be used for testing.

Chronic: Refers to a recurring, persistent condition that does not get healed completely. These include conditions such as heart disease and diabetes.

Contusion - A bruise.

Defibrillator - This refers to an electric device that uses electric shock to restore the normal body functions of a patient. Such devices are used when a person faints, or the heart fails.

Edema - Refers to swelling of body parts due to the collection of fluids. This commonly occurs in people suffering from arthritis.

Embolism - A situation where an artery blocks due to blood clotting. This can lead to high blood pressure and, in some instances, is cause for a heart attack.

Epidermis - The outer layer of the skin.

Fracture - Broken bone or cartilage. The medical term for a broken bone in a patient.

Gland - An organ or tissue that produces and secretes fluids that serve a specific function.

Hypertension - High blood pressure.

Inpatient: Refers to a patient that must be admitted into the hospital for inward treatments. Opposite of outpatient or patients that get treated and go back home.

Intravenous: A fluid or medication that is delivered through the vein to the body.

Malignant - Indicates the presence of cancer in cells.

Outpatient - A patient who receives the care and goes back home without having to spend a night at the hospital.

Prognosis - Refers to the expected outcome of disease treatment. The prognosis simply refers to the journey the patient will take towards recovery.

Relapse - Return of disease or symptoms after a patient has recovered. The reoccurrence of the symptoms of a condition after a patient had been treated and well recovered.

Sutures - Stitches, which are used to join tissues together as they heal. Refers to the stitches used to hold tissue together when a patient has an open wound or when they undergo surgery.

Transplant - The removal of an organ or tissue from one body that is implanted into another. This refers to the removal of an organ from one body and transfer to another. It might be removed from the patient's body and used on the same patient, or it might be removed from an organ donor and transferred to the patient.

Vaccine - A substance that stimulates antibody production to provide immunity against disease. A substance that is administered to healthy individuals to stimulate antibody production in order to enhance immunity. Vaccines help the body fight against specific infections.

Zoonotic disease - A disease that is transmissible from animals to humans and vice-versa.

Medical Prefixes and Suffixes

Medical terms follow the same structural rules all language does, including using prefixes and suffixes. You probably know some of these from words outside of medicine.

A-, an- Lack of or without.

-ation - a process

Dys- - abnormal, difficult, or painful.

-ectomy - Surgical removal of something.

-ismus - a spasm or contraction.

-itis - inflammation.

-lysis - decomposition, destruction, or breaking down.

Macro- Large in size.

Melan/o- Black or dark in color.

Micro- small in size.

-ology - The study of something.

-osis - indicates something is abnormal.

-otomy - to cut into.

-pathy - disease or disease process.

-plasty - surgical repair.

Poly- Many

Pseudo - False or deceptive, usually in regard to appearance.

Retro- Behind or backward.

Medical Root Words

Cardi/o: This is a term often used when referring to anything related to the heart.

Derm/a/o, dermat/o: The abbreviation term or format is used when referring to the skin. A dermatologist is a skin doctor.

Encephal/o: This abbreviation is used when referring to the brain.

Gastr/o: The term gastric is used to mean the stomach. You have probably heard about gastrointestinal infections.

Hemat/o: The short form Hemat refers to anything to do with blood.

My/o - Related to the muscles.

Oste/o: The term Osteo is used in reference to the bone or bone structure.

Pulmon/o: Refers to the lungs and can be used when referring to lung conditions.

Rhin/o - Related to the nose.

Sclerosis - Hard or hardening.

Stasis: Refers to the stopping of the flow of body fluids such as blood,

Therm/o: The term therm is very common and is used in reference to many aspects when referring to body temperature.

Medical Abbreviations and Acronyms

There are many more medical terms than those listed below. These should be sufficient for preppers.

ALS - Advanced Life Support.

Bl wk - Blood work.

BMI - Body mass index - a measure of body fat based on height and weight.

BP - Blood pressure.

CPR - Cardiopulmonary resuscitation, a lifesaving technique that's also called mouth-to-mouth resuscitation.

C-spine - Cervical spine - these are the 7 bones in the

neck region of the spine.

DNR - Do not resuscitate - a medical order indicating providers shouldn't perform CPR.

ED/ER - Emergency department or emergency room.

EKG - Electrocardiogram - a way of monitoring the heart and testing for problems.

HDL-C - High-density lipoprotein cholesterol, often called "bad" cholesterol.

HR - heart rate, expressed as beats per minute.

LDL-C - Low-density lipoprotein cholesterol, often called "bad" cholesterol.

Lytes - Electrolytes.

NICU - Neonatal intensive care unit, a special unit that cares for premature infants.

OR - operating room, where surgeries are performed

Pre-op - Pre-operative.

Psych - Refers to psychiatry or the psychiatric ward.

PT - physical therapy, a type of treatment to help patients move and feel better.

Rx - Prescription, usually for medication, but can also signify another treatment.

Stat - Immediately.

How to Deal with Chronic Conditions

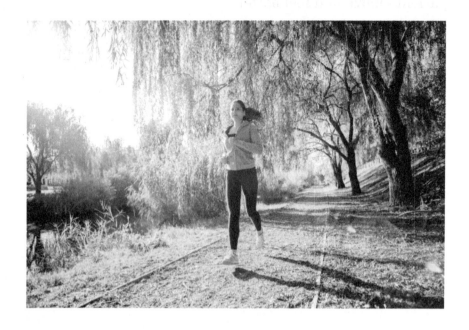

When you are planning for doomsday medical care, you must think about chronic conditions. You may not be suffering from a chronic condition yourself, but your skills may be very helpful in dealing with such situations. The idea of dealing with chronic conditions in an SHFT situation can be scary in itself, but you must gather the courage to be able to survive the hardest times of your life.

What if you're a prepper who has a chronic condition?

It can be difficult to survive in a world that has few resources available if you have a chronic condition or disability, but there are ways to survive. We'll discuss those in this chapter.

What is a Chronic Condition?

First, let's define what a chronic condition is. A chronic condition is one that always exists - it doesn't come and go based on certain environmental factors. These could include conditions like:

Physical disabilities	Arthritis	Endometriosis
Asthma	Celiac disease	Inflammatory bowel disease
Hashimoto's thyroiditis	Lupus	Lyme disease
Chronic fatigue syndrome	Fibromyalgia	Rheumatoid arthritis
Diabetes	Adrenal fatigue	Mental health problems

Hypertension	Autoimmune disorders	Cancer

It's not a comprehensive list, but it gives you an idea of some of the conditions we're talking about in this section.

People with chronic conditions may not be able to do everything they'd like to, but they can still be a big asset to their community. They can still help manage disasters, plant a garden, preserve food, and learn skills. They may need to do things a little differently than folks who don't have the same problems. Each individual has their own limitations. You have to improve what you can and improvise what you can't. Here are a few tips for preppers with a chronic illness or disability:

Be Personally Prepared

You should be aware of this if you're taking medication or need any kind of special supplies or equipment. If medical supplies run out, even a low-level crisis can be major. Your doctor can prescribe your medication several months ahead of time, and you can get your refills a month sooner - you can cite the fact that it is cheaper to buy in larger quantities, and it will save you money on your pharmacy's end.

Not having important medication or supplies on hand means that someone you care about may have to put themselves at risk to get more for you in a situation in which they'd be safer staying at home. It means that you may need medical intervention when no one is available. It's easier just to stock up ahead of time. If your dosage is changed, continue to fill your previous lower prescription to add to your stockpile.

You need to understand your medical condition.

Most people with a chronic illness already know that they have to become their own physician to some degree, especially when it's a lesser understood illness.

Be aware of danger signs, behavior changes you can make, ways to relieve symptoms without having to take your medications, and dietary changes you can make. You also need to understand the behaviors and activities that make your condition worse and avoid them if possible. Stock up on things that will make you more comfortable, and keep reference information at hand in hard copy format.

Stay as close to your regular diet as possible.

Stocking up on food for an emergency means choosing foods that make you feel better. Especially if you control some of your symptoms with diet, an emergency is not the time to consume foods that will increase inflammation or cause digestive problems.

For example, if you need to maintain a low-carb diet to manage your condition, you'll want to avoid eating rice and pasta-based meals. They'll make you sick very fast. However, if you're a vegan, suddenly gnawing on jerky or creamy soups won't make you feel well either. This goes back to the prepper adage, "Eat what you store and store what you eat."

Make accommodations.

You can still do things even if you can't do them the same way everyone else does them. The following adjustments might work for you, or they might spark your creative juices:

Raised beds should be built to a comfortable height. They make gardening easier since you don't have to bend over. If you're in a wheelchair, make sure there's enough space between the beds and that the surface is smooth and clean.

Invest in a gardening stool with handles to provide support when getting up and down. This can also be used in other places

Use smaller containers when you repackage your food. Instead of 5-gallon buckets, use one-gallon buckets if you are experiencing pain, mobility issues, or strength issues

The same goes for stored water. You won't want to deal with 5-gallon water jugs, so pick 1-gallon instead.

If you're paralyzed or can't walk long distances, figure out how you could make a trek if you needed to.

Use a reach grabber to reach things on high shelves instead of climbing on something. You don't want to risk getting injured on top of everything else.

Use jar openers and bucket openers if you have less strength. Pick up these two things now to make your life easier.

Make your home user-friendly with grab handles and other mobility aids.

Exercise if you can.

Nearly all health conditions can benefit from moderate exercise, modified for your needs. In an emergency, the better your fitness level, the better off you'll be. If you can, walk every day. Make sure you are strengthening your muscles, cardiovascular system, and mobility at home if you can't walk. These could include:

Shoulder retractions: Straighten your back and contract your abdominal muscles to support the back muscles. Hold your hands at shoulder level at a 90-degree angle, fingers curved as if you were gripping bicycle handles. Stretch out your arms as far as you can without locking your joints. Pull your arms back until they are just slightly behind your torso, squeezing together your shoulder blades as you do so. Then repeat the motion.

Chest squeeze: Hold a medicine ball, rubber ball, or balloon at chest level, squeezing the ball between your hands to contract the chest muscles while sitting up straight. Continue to squeeze the ball through the entire movement, pushing it forward until your elbows are almost straight. Slowly pull the ball back and repeat.

Toe taps: Sit up straight with abs engaged and feet flat on the ground. Tilt your toes up towards the ceiling and then back down to the floor. Repeat several times. To make it more difficult, raise one leg in the air, so it's straight out in front of you, keeping the other foot flat on the floor. Tilt your toes up and down several times. Lower the foot back down to the floor and repeat with the other leg.

Knee lifts: Sit up straight with the abs engaged and feet flat on the ground. Slowly lift your right leg, bending your knee in a marching motion. Lift your leg as high as possible comfortably, then lower your foot back down to the floor and repeat with the other leg. Continue to repeat this motion, alternating legs.

Tummy twist: Sit up straight with your abs engaged and your feet flat on the ground. Position your arms at a 90-degree angle with your forearms extended in front of you and elbows at your sides. Rotate your upper torso to the left while twisting at the waist as far as you are comfortable. Rotate back to the center and repeat the motion to the right. During the movement, imagine sucking your belly button towards your spine and keeping your lower body completely still.

Captain's chair: Sit up straight and grab the front edge of your seat with both hands. Slowly lift both of your feet off the floor, bending your knees towards your chest as you do, lifting as high as you comfortably can. Squeeze your abs at the top of the movement, and lower both feet back to the floor. Be careful not to raise your legs past a comfortable position. If you can only raise your feet a few inches off the floor to start, that's fine.

Side bend stretch: Sit up tall, abdominal muscles contracted and hips facing squarely forward. Extend your left arm toward the ceiling, keeping the inside of your upper arm very close to your ear. Hold your left arm in that position, and slowly bend your entire upper body to the right, making a "C" shape. To make it more intense, reach your right arm towards the floor. Hold the stretch for 5-15 seconds. Slowly move back to center and repeat on the other side.

Have a plan.

Consider what happened to many wheelchair-bound and elderly people when the levee broke after Hurricane Katrina. They drowned because they didn't have a plan in place. That didn't have to happen.

If you have decreased mobility for any reason, now is the time to make a plan. Bugging in should almost always be your plan A, but if the situation calls for a plan B, how will you bug out? This is going to be different for everyone, but it's important to figure it out before an epic disaster gives you five minutes to be out the door.

Let others know about your condition. If you're in a community, let others know about your condition or limitations so they can help get you to safety. Let them know what kind of condition you have and what they'll need to do if a disaster strikes.

Online shopping made the world a lot bigger for people with chronic illnesses and disabilities. If you have mobility or fatigue issues, going out for a long day of stock-up shopping probably sounds like torture. Start buying your provisions online and get them delivered to your door. You can often find better deals online than you can in your own area, which makes online shopping an even bigger win. But even grocery stores and pharmacies now deliver in many places, which can be a bonus when you're making larger purchases because you don't have to get them in from the car.

You can weigh this against concerns about OPSEC and privacy, but so many people shop online these days that the mailman won't think much about a few Amazon packages here and there. Break up your purchases instead of getting 50 boxes delivered in the span of a week, and it won't even be notable to your delivery person.

Focus on knowledge and skills.

Even though you won't be out there working after some apocalyptic event, you can still be a valuable member of the group. What kind of knowledge and skills do you have, or what can you learn that will help others? Not only will this help your family, but it often can be bartered to others in exchange for the things you can't do. Here are a few ideas:

Herbalism

Foraging

Food preservation

Sewing/Mending

Medical knowledge

Repairing

Old-fashioned skills - how did people complete
everyday tasks before the days of convenience and
electricity? Your knowledge and abilities in this area can
be invaluable.

Find a community.

This isn't always easy or possible, but if you can at all,
find a like-minded community of people who are on the
same page with you. Maybe this will be your family, or it
could be friends and neighbors. Regardless, it's hard to
survive alone, even if you're in good health. If you have
limitations, the help of other people will be essential. Just
make sure you have something to offer them in return,
whether it's supplies or knowledge.

Be prepared to protect yourself.

As horrible as this sounds, some people will see your disability or ill health and consider you an easy target. We can't always wait for 911 to rescue us, so it's important that you can rescue yourself.

A firearm is the best way to do this. If you don't know how to shoot, find a gun range that you can practice at and work with an instructor who can help you make accommodations for your disability or lack of strength. A good instructor can help you choose a firearm that will work best with your limitations. Remember, you need to continue practicing this skill regularly. If someone sees you as a target, you have no option but to protect yourself.

Managing Common Conditions

Diabetes

Diabetes is a delicate condition that usually stays with a person for life. Although there are some claims of full recovery, most people who suffer from diabetes have to deal with the condition for life. In our modern medical setup, diabetes patients are given drugs that help balance blood sugar levels or enhance pancreas performance. They also follow doctors' guidelines on a diet to avoid chances where blood sugar levels spike.

In an SHFT situation, there may be no foods to help you monitor your intake. At such a time, the chances of blood sugar spikes are very high. As a result, you should be prepared for the first aid steps you should take to stabilize the patient before taking other steps.

When a person suffering from diabetes experiences a blood sugar spike, they may faint. If a person faints as a result of blood sugar reduction, give them something sweet to eat. In most cases, people are given glucose or sugar to stabilize their blood sugars. Once the person regains consciousness, make sure you take steps that will help the patient remain stable. These steps include administering diabetic drugs.

The best diabetes drug is insulin. If a person suffers from diabetes, their main problem is low insulin levels. However, the treatments for diabetes type 2 vary widely from the treatments for diabetes type 1. When shopping for your diabetes drugs, make sure you know the types of diabetes you intend to treat. As a precautionary measure, it is recommended that you stock up on all types of diabetes drugs.

There are many types of diabetes drugs you may stock up in your prepper's pantry. Among the common diabetes drugs are glimepiride (Amaryl, glimepiride-pioglitazone (Duetact), glimepiride-rosiglitazone (Avandaryl), gliclazide and glipizide (Glucotrol).

Heart Disease

There are seven types of diseases that can be classified as heart disease. They include

Coronary Artery Disease (CAD)

Heart Arrhythmias

Heart Failure

Heart Valve Disease

Pericardial Disease

Cardiomyopathy (Heart Muscle Disease)

Congenital Heart Disease

Each of these conditions can only be treated by ensuring that your heart is in a well-functioning state. More often than not, the best treatment for heart disease is exercising and observing your diet. Even so, it is important to have some medications around. There are medications that generally help with all types of heart conditions. These are mainly blood-thinning drugs such as Apixaban (Eliquis), Dabigatran (Pradaxa), Dalteparin (Fragmin), Edoxaban (Savaysa) and Enoxaparin (Lovenox).

You may also want to try stocking some statins such as atorvastatin (Lipitor), lovastatin (Altoprev), fluvastatin (Lescol XL), pitavastatin (Livaloatorvastatin (Lipitor), lovastatin (Altoprev), pitavastatin (Livalo) and fluvastatin (Lescol XL). These drugs are responsible for reducing inhibitors found in high cholesterol products.

The other types of heart disease medications you should consider stockpiling are beta-blockers, angiotensin-converting enzymes (ACE), calcium channel blockers, and angiotensin 2 receptor blockers, among others. These drugs mostly require a doctor's prescription, but by following some of our suggested tricks, you may be able to obtain most of the heart disease drugs.

High Blood Pressure

The other condition you should be ready to deal with is high blood pressure. Any person can experience a blood pressure spike, especially when anxious. If the situation is not handled well, further complications are likely to ensue. It is good to have some skills that can help you deal with high blood pressure.

The first step you should take when a person is experiencing high pressure is to try and calm them down. This might be quite difficult, but it is achievable. Let them lay on the ground in an open place and loosen their clothes for easy breathing.

In terms of medication, you should only administer drugs after the patient gets out of immediate danger. Once the patient is out of danger and quite stable, administer any of these drugs according to instructions. The main drugs used in the US are Amlodipine besylate (Norvasc, Lotrel), Clevidipine (Cleviprex), Diltiazem hydrochloride (Cardizem CD, Cardizem SR, Dilacor XR, Tiazac), Felodipine (Plendil), Isradipine (DynaCirc, DynaCirc CR), and Nicardipine (Cardene SR).

Arthritis

Arthritis can be a terrible condition for anyone who does not have access to medical assistance. Given that this is a long-term chronic condition, you should stock up sufficient drugs to help keep it in control for as long as possible.

There are various remedies that can be used to help arthritis patients in case you do not have access to medical help. The main remedy is heating the joints with a hot pad. The joint pains caused by arthritis can be reduced significantly by heating the joints with drugs or submerging the affected area in hot water.

According to the Arthritis Foundation, cayenne pepper can also be used to reduce the pain caused by arthritis. Cayenne is an anti-inflammatory and works well in reducing joint swelling and pain. Other types of peppers are also highly recommended for arthritis patients.

However, instead of waiting too long just to start risking with herbs, it is better to pack sufficient arthritis drugs. Currently, there are several drugs approved for the treatment and management of arthritis. The drugs to look out for are Methotrexate (Rheumatrex, Trexall),

Hydroxychloroquine (Plaquenil), Sulfasalazine (Azulfidine), Leflunomide (Arava), and Tumor Necrosis Factor Inhibitors.

Cancer

The other chronic condition you want to think about is cancer. There are different types of cancer that show up at different levels. The only problem with cancer is that it comes in different types, and diagnosis is quite difficult. It is almost impossible to prepare for an SHFT event in terms of cancer. However, for those who are already on cancer treatment, it is advisable to stock up as many drugs as possible for your treatment. In case anything happens and you are unable to access medical care, you should have enough drugs to keep you going.

Since there are different drugs administered at different levels of cancer treatments, I will not give you a list of drugs to buy. Make sure you get a hint of what is necessary from your current treatments.

HIV

The other condition that requires care in an SHFT situation is HIV. Any person suffering from HIV should always have extra stock of ARVs just in case something happens. If you are on HIV medication, make arrangements to get more suppliers of the drugs in advance.

Since HIV is a sexually transmitted infection, make sure you also stock up sufficient sexual protection products. During hard times, people find consolation in intimacy. People get intimate even with strangers just to escape the trauma of whatever is happening around them. In such circumstances, having a sufficient supply of protection such as condoms might be necessary. You do not want to get infected at a time when there is no medical care around.

How to Stay Safe When Providing Medical Care

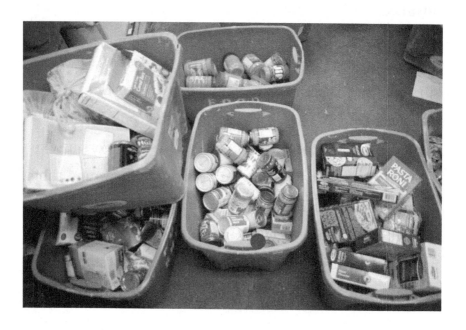

In a situation where you have to provide medical care to someone, make sure you take care of your own safety first. It is even more dangerous to lose the only person who can provide medical care in an SHFT situation. During the COVID-19 peak, many doctors were lost to the disease. All the doctors lost left a huge gap that made the fight against the disease difficult. The first step in the fight against any type of condition is to protect your soldiers. If you are the best bet for those who need medical help, make sure you are safe.

If you're in the middle of an SHTF event and have had to find a home somewhere out away from where you used to live, it can be difficult to know how to stay safe when providing medical care. In this section, I'll provide some information on how to do that.

There are different levels of safety to consider in an SHFT situation. We may look at health safety and safety against physical threats such as bullets in a war situation. To keep yourself safe, here are some guidelines to observe:

Always Wear Protective Gear When Handling Patients

Make sure you wear protective gear every time you come in contact with a patient. Even when the patient is being transported, make sure you have your mask, apron, and gloves on. These wearables go a long way in reducing potential risks that may occur if you get in contact with a contaminated surface.

In a war situation, wear bulletproof clothing. You should make sure you protect yourself at all costs. You may want to wear protective gear for war situations.

These include bulletproof vests, helmets, and other necessary wearables. The wearables may help save your life in case you are targeted by a gunshot.

Evacuate Patients at the Least Risky Times

Patient evacuations should not be a reason for you to lose your life. In a patient evacuation, you should ensure that all the required medical standards are met to keep the patient safe but also to keep you safe. When you evacuate a patient, always make sure the patient is made to lay down facing up. The patient should be as comfortable as possible. All supporting necessities should be on hand. These may include painkillers, oxygen support was possible, among others. You also want to bring along your equipment to monitor the patient along the way.

In a war, the situation makes sure you evacuate your patients when it is safe. There are no times that are absolutely safe, but you will be sure to find safe hours in a day. During hours when waring functions retreat to regroup, you have a chance of moving your patient a lot more safely. Of course, safety is never guaranteed in such times, but you have to choose the least risky situations.

Wear a Humanitarian Badge if Possible

One of the sure ways to remain safe in an SHFT situation is to put on a humanitarian badge. A person wearing a humanitarian badge can be spared even by the warring factions. This is because humanitarian groups are given a way to offer assistance where possible. Both sides know that they can use the services of a doctor at any time. They will not easily harm a humanitarian doctor trying to give help.

Set up a Survival Sick Room

Obviously, we can no longer use modern medical facilities, but it's still possible to set up a survival sick room to protect those who are injured. We may have to go back to doing things the way they were done in the 19th century, but now we know more about medications and hygiene than we did then, so we can use that knowledge when setting up a survival sick room.

If you're out in the wilderness and haven't found a

building or place to use for shelter, you can set up a tent if you have one. This helps minimize the chances of diseases being transmitted to others in the community or area where you've set up camp.

If you don't have a tent or a place you can set up as a sick room, use a makeshift barrier, such as a sheet of plastic, to separate the sick people from the healthy ones. If you know a disaster is coming but it hasn't arrived yet, set up a barrier or sick room now, so you're prepared when the shit does hit the fan.

Furnishings in sick rooms should be minimal. You should have a work surface, exam area, and some spaces for beds. If the weather is mild, some of the beds can be outside, as long as you can provide shade with a canopy or something else. Try to provide hard surfaces instead of upholstered ones because the cloth can hold disease-causing organisms. You may even want to cover bedding in plastic. The more areas you can disinfect easily, the better.

Also, make sure you have a way to eliminate waste products for bedridden patients, even if you just use a 5-gallon bucket and some bleach. Remember that urine begins to break down after a few days and will start smelling like ammonia. If you can, dump it outdoors in a pit or gravel bed because the ammonia in urine will kill grass, trees, crops, and other vegetation.

As for feces, a toilet you can flush with buckets of water is your best option. If this isn't available, though, you'll have to use a bucket and lid. You can throw any toilet paper or feminine hygiene products in there as well, so you don't mix them with your regular trash. Be sure to add a little dry material after each use as well, such as wood ashes, sawdust, or dried grass. Dried material helps reduce the smell, along with a splash of chlorine bleach.

You'll also want to have a bucket to use to create a compost pit. You can dump the contents of your waste bucket in this. When you make it, be sure to put layers of grass and/or leftovers from vegetables, such as pieces of uneaten carrot, or peelings from fruits or vegetables, into the compost bin and turn it regularly. It takes about three months for food to compost and requires regular maintenance.

You should use containers with lids for dirty sick room items. You should also set up a station near the entrance of the sickroom for masks, gloves, gowns and aprons, or other personal protective items you may have gathered before the SHTF event. You should also have a basin with water, soap, rubbing alcohol, and peroxide. If you have thermometers, dip them in alcohol to keep them disinfected.

Other supplies you'll want to have in your sick room include:

Gauze: This is used to cover wounds, so they stay clean. It's available in sponges of different sizes or as strips that can be wrapped around a wound. Place the gauze sponge over the wound, and then wrap the gauze strips around it to keep the sponge in place.

Tourniquets: These are used to stop bleeding when an injury is so bad that a bandage alone isn't stopping it.

Other dressings: These could include non-adherent pads, non-adherent wet dressings, foam dressings, calcium alginates, hydrogel dressings, and transparent dressings.

You'll also need sets of sheets, towels, pillows, and other items used in a sick room. Keep these separate from the items for the healthy members of your group.

Your sick room will need to be cleaned thoroughly every day, so you'll also want to have cleaning items in your sick room. Hard surfaces should be cleaned with soap and water or other solutions such as a 1:10 beach to water solution. Don't forget to disinfect any doorknobs, sinks, toilets, counters, or toys in the sick area.

How to Transport Sick and Injured People in an SHTF Situation

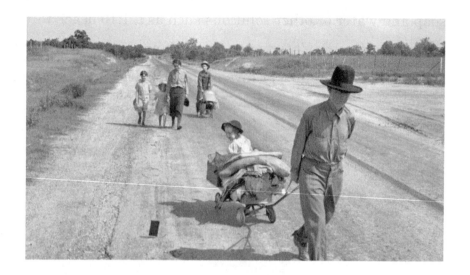

What if you become sick or injured, or you're with someone who becomes sick or injured, and you're not near the sick room? There's no ambulance available, so how do you get there? We'll discuss how to transport sick or injured people here.

Transport Using Materials You Find

If you don't have access to stretchers or other things that would be used to transport people in a non-crisis situation, transport using anything you can find. This could include things like:

Blankets

Inside doors

Ironing boards

You can use folded over rope, blankets, or parachute cords as handholds for the blankets, doors, or boards to use to transport the sick or injured person.

Something else you can use to transport an injured person is a chair. The injured person would sit in the chair. One of the transporters would stand behind the chair and tilt it back; the other would grab the chair in front. Both people would then lift and carry the chair. The second transporter can face the victim for short distances, but for longer distances, it's better if both face forward.

If you don't have a sturdy backboard or a chair to use to transport sick or injured people, you can also use blankets or clothing to transport them. You can do this using one, two or four people.

One-Person Blanket Pull

If you're alone with the victim and can't wait for help to arrive, place a blanket under them. Grasp the blanket with both hands at one end. Let your forearms cradle their head. Use your legs to pull instead of the back, so you don't injure yourself. You can also drag the victim by the shoulder of their shirt or jacket. Grasp the back of the clothing under their shoulders and use your legs to pull. If it's done right, your arms should cradle the head.

Two-Person Blanket Stretcher

You can easily make a litter using two long poles or sticks that are about 6 to 7 feet long and two to four inches thick.

Lay the blanket flat on the ground and place the two sticks on top, so the blanket is divided into thirds. Fold both of the outer thirds over the sticks, back toward the middle. Once that's done, the patient's weight will keep the blanket and folds in place during transport.

You can also use two jackets with buttons to create a stretcher. Two buttoned jackets should be used, preferably the ones on the rescuers. First, the transporter grasps the litter poles, then the second takes off the jacket by pulling it inside out. The jacket automatically moves onto the poles, forming a bed for the stretcher. When the transporters reverse roles, a second shirt or jacket is inserted into the pole. This method should only be used if the weather is nice enough that the rescuers can tolerate not wearing jackets or shirts during transport.

Four-Person Blanket Stretcher

This one is useful if you have four people helping the sick or injured person. Even if you have no backboard, a blanket or sturdy poncho can help move an injured person. Just place the victim on the stretched-out blanket and then roll the sides inward to form handholds for the four people to lift and carry the victim.

Transporting Using No Materials

What if you have nothing to transport a sick or injured person with except your own muscles? It can still be done. We'll explain how to do it in this section.

Using a Three-Person Team

If you have three people available to help transport the injured person, you can form a "hammock" that will make it easier to lift and transport them. With this method, rescuers kneel on both sides of the victim. You'll reach under the person to grasp the wrist of the person across from you. The people at each end will use one hand to support the head and feet of the person being moved. Upon command, rescuers will get on one knee and then stand.

Sometimes it is necessary to get a patient onto a higher level than a stretcher, such as a gurney or operating table. In this case, you can use the three-person carry to lift the victim short distances. The transporters kneel on one knee and roll the patient on his side, so he is facing the rescuers. They then lift him onto their knees, and they stand up on command. The transporters hold the victim on their chests, and they all start evacuation on the same foot.

Using a Two-Person Team

When it's just you and one other assistant, you can do a

few different things. If your casualty is conscious and can hold on to your shoulders, you can make a four-handed seat with interlocked wrists. With all four wrists interlocked in a square, a wider, more stable seat is formed. If one of the rescuers needs a free hand, three wrists can form a triangular seat.

Use the two-handed seat method. This is useful for victims who might be less alert. Each rescuer interlocks one wrist to form a seat and uses the other arm to grasp his partner's shoulder. This forms the back support. All versions start with the transporters squatting on either side of the victim, using their legs to lift instead of their backs.

The crutch method allows a conscious patient to walk using the rescuers as a pair of crutches. Each rescuer grabs a wrist and puts the crook of the arm on the back of their neck and over the shoulder, with the other arm around the victim's waist. The patient can then stand with assistance. If they're unconscious, the waistband or belt can be pulled to help lift the casualty, with their legs dragging behind as you move.

The fore-and-aft technique can work well as a long-distance transport method for conscious or unconscious victims. The first rescuer is behind the victim and puts his arms under the shoulders of the victim lying on his back, and locks his hands around the chest. The second rescuer, facing front toward the victim's feet, uses both arms to grasp underneath each knee. It's more comfortable if the taller transporter is at the patient's head.

One Person Transport

Sometimes it's just you and the victim, and you have no equipment. There are still ways you can evacuate a patient.

Use a fireman's carry. While you're squatting or kneeling, grasp the person's right wrist with your left hand and drape it over your shoulders. As you keep your back straight, hold them by the right thigh with your right hand. As you stand up, use your legs. Their torso should be over your back, and their right thigh should rest on your right shoulder. The left arm and leg of the patient should hang behind your back if you've done it correctly. Make sure the patient is in the right position so that you feel the least strain.

You can also use the pack-strap carry if you are the sole rescuer. Cross both arms across your chest while facing the patient behind and behind you. Lift the patient by using your legs and back muscles while squatting. Lean forward slightly so that they are resting on your hips, and then lift them.

How to Perform an Emergency Amputation and Deal with Severed Body Parts

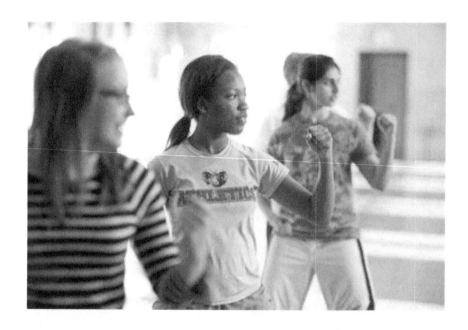

If a person injures some part of their body so badly that they won't be able to survive unless it's amputated, then you have no choice but to amputate it. But how do you perform an emergency amputation in an SHTF situation? We'll discuss that in this section.

First, you need to understand this should only be done if there's an immediate risk to their life if the affected limb isn't amputated. This could mean that the patient would die before they reached a doctor if the limb wasn't amputated - and in an SHTF situation, who knows if there will be a doctor available?

Amputation Procedures

If you have to amputate a body part, follow these steps:

1. Make a circular incision through the skin and deep tissue at the lowest possible level and let that layer retract.

2. Divide the exposed muscle bundles at the new level of the skin edge. They will then promptly retract, exposing the bone.

3. Place upward pressure on the proximal muscle stump and take out the bone at a higher level. The wound will look like an inverted cone.

4. Isolate and clamp the blood vessels, ligate them, and apply bone wax to the end of the bone to prevent oozing.

5. Take out major nerves at the highest level possible.

6. Put a layer of fine mesh gauze over the wound and pack the recess with fluffed gauze. Place stocking over the stump and wrap it with Ace wraps. Use compression decreasing proximally, and apply 5-6 pounds of traction. Continued traction will cause the skin to close over the stump.

FAQs of Severe Wounds

Can you use Superglue to close a wound?

Yes and no. Superglue will close wounds the same way medical adhesive does; however it's not sterile, and different brands have different preservatives, which can be harmful to injured tissue. It probably won't be a problem for small wounds, but the potential for toxicity goes up when large amounts are used.

Should you use a tourniquet?

You should only use a tourniquet if all other methods to stop bleeding have failed. This is because tourniquets can damage tissue when they're used correctly. Tourniquets have to be tight in order to work correctly. When they're removed, the resulting tissue damage causes swelling, which is called edema.

What should you do with severed body parts?

If you lose a body part in an SHTF situation, unless you've got a good hospital/sick room set up, chances are it's not going to be re-attached. The best thing to do with a severed body part is to bury it. Gravesites have been set up in the past for severed body parts. In an SHTF situation, when you have to have a body part amputated, and there's no hospital available to dispose of the limb, it might not be a bad idea to set up a gravesite for severed body parts.

How to Deal with the Dead

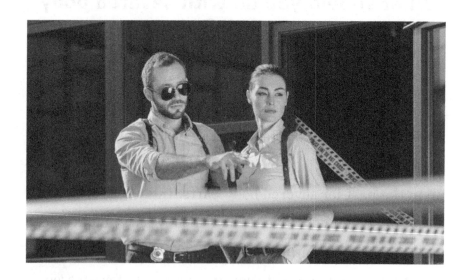

What happens if someone dies in an SHTF situation? You can't give them the type of burial and service they would likely otherwise receive, but you can still bury them and find ways to deal with their passing.

It is normal for people to die, especially where they are being treated. The sooner you get in touch with this reality, the better. If you are afraid of death or dead bodies, you should not move anywhere to a medical center camp. In any situation, people may pass away even in your own hands. It is important to prepare yourself for such realities when preparing for an SHFT event.

General Concerns for the Dead

You need to have an idea of how to deal with dead bodies when you are in such a situation. Remember that dead bodies are not being handled by the government in an SHFT situation. There are no mortuaries or funeral homes. Those who are responsible for handling dead bodies are the closest friends and family members. It is also vital to remember that dead bodies can be hazardous in spreading disease. You must have an idea of how to handle dead bodies in different situations. This includes how to burry, dress, and preserve them, among other factors.

1. Know how and why they died. If it's because of injuries, your main concern should be your safety. The cause of their injuries could still be around if it's another human being, animals, insects, or a natural disaster. If the person died because of illness, make sure the disease doesn't spread.

2. After someone close to us dies, they should receive a proper burial. Before you bury them, look at your situation and make sure you're not in immediate danger.

3. Move the body away from water because human remains can contaminate drinking water. If the deceased person died of an illness, be careful when touching the body. Use gloves or something else you can find to create a barrier between you and possible diseases.

4. Ensure that everyone in your group helps you bury the body. Try to dig a hole that's at least six feet deep when possible.

5. Take care of yourself. It's not easy to handle death. The pain of losing someone can cause you to think illogically and put you at further risk. So after someone dies, take care of yourself. Take time to mourn and help others through it as well. Everyone mourns differently, so support everyone around you.

Dead Body Preservation Techniques

In modern-day body preservation, two main techniques are used. They either use refrigeration or chemical preservation. Large morgues combine chemical preservation and refrigeration. In the event that morgues are no longer functional, you should be in a position to preserve bodies. In most cases, there will be no time to bury bodies, but preservation might give you a chance to bury your loved ones well.

Unfortunately, in an SHFT situation, refrigeration is almost impractical. You need large fridges to keep the bodies cool. In a most disastrous situation, even fridges will not be available. In this case, you will be left with chemical preservation. For this reason, I will recommend that you also get some dead body preservation chemicals when stocking up your medical prepper's pantry.

The chemical formaldehyde is injected into the dead body to change the tissue structure such that bacteria cannot eat on them. This is one of the easiest and most recommended ways of preservation. If you have the chemical, simply use it to inject the dead body. Normally, the body is injected when it is still quite fresh. As soon as a person dies, the body should be washed and injected with the chemical. This helps it to circulate well into the dead body. Further, it prevents bacteria spread, which can be quite difficult to stop once it has started.

In case you do not have access to refrigeration or chemicals, you will have to turn to alternative preservation methods. Traditionally bodies were not preserved in the fridge or with chemicals. People had to find ways of dealing with dead bodies that can still be used today. These ways include natural refrigeration techniques such as charcoal refrigeration.

Charcoal Refrigeration

This is a method of dead body preservation where the body is laid over cold charcoal. The charcoal is sprinkled with water to make it cool. Cool charcoal absorbs heat from the dead body keeping it cool for several days. Although this is an ancient technique, it can be used in a situation where access to modern refrigeration is limited.

Covered Floor Refrigeration

You may also use concrete floor refrigeration. In this approach, the body is laid on a cool concrete floor. The floor should be quite dry but very cool. This might give the body some time to stay fresh while you plan for the way forward.

Besides these techniques, you should always keep the dead body clean. Put it in a cool, dry place while you look for other options on how to handle the body.

How to Prevent Getting Infected by Dead Bodies

In the COVID-19 scenario, dead bodies were required to be buried within 24 hours in most places. Furthermore, the bodies were only handled by experts. Those handling the body were dressed in special gear, covering them from top to bottom. Such can be the scenario in different situations.

If the case is of a dangerous infectious disease, it is vital to use protective gear while handling dead bodies. Dead bodies that pose a risk of infecting people with a dangerous disease should be disposed of as soon as possible. You should not spend much time with such a body. In case of a contagious disease, the body should be disposed of within one day of death.

To ensure that a contagious body does not spread the disease to others, it should be wrapped in plastic bags immediately after death. Wrap the body and put the body in a dead body's room. All the belongings and clothing used by the dead should either be sterilized or disposed of in the required manner. Do not allow anyone to use such clothing and bedding before they are well sanitized or sterilized based on the medical information available at the time.

Burying the Dead Body

Burying a dead body should not be a big issue if you have attended a burial before. In a situation where there are no funeral homes to handle the dead, it may be your role to ensure that the dead are buried. If the dead bodies are highly dangerous, you want to make sure they are buried as soon as possible. When it comes to burying dead bodies, there are many options available. You could choose to bury them in shallow graves, let the body alone, or cremate them.

In such a tough situation, you should be ready to make the decisions yourself. It is sometimes difficult to decide what you will do with the body before we can know the type of situation you will be dealing with. However, in a situation where you will be dealing with a dangerous dead body, just prepare a shallow grave and bury the dead. Ideally, make sure the body is wrapped in a piece of clothing. If you are lucky enough to access a coffin, you may use one. Ideally, bodies should be buried in designated sites such as the cemetery. However, sometimes you may fail to access a cemetery. In such a situation, burying the dead, even in your backyard, may not be a big deal.

Ideally, dead bodies should be buried with other dead bodies unless otherwise necessary. If you do not have anything hindering you from burying your dead, make sure they are laid to rest within three days. If you have other constraints, you may want to try the above-mentioned preservation techniques to see how long you can hold the case.

In the case where burial is not possible, cremation should be a possibility. This is especially true in the cases where the dead body carries a big risk of causing infections to the community. In such a situation, people may turn to cremation to destroy any chances of spreading the disease within the community.

Finally, when someone gets injured or dies after an SHTF event, the one thing you need to remember is you did the best you could. It's not your fault. What's important is that you focus on your own survival as you go forward.

FAQs on Medical Necessities for a Prepper

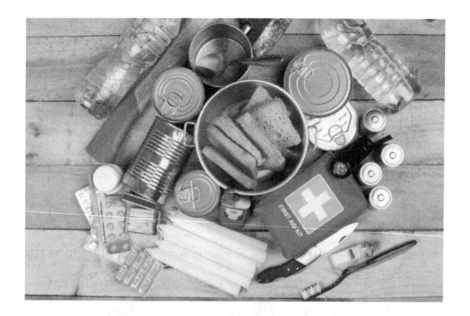

Q. Must I store all types of medication?

The type of medication you store is entirely dependent on your capacity and intentions. It would be ideal to have all types of mediation in your prepper's pantry. The only problem is that you could not accumulate all the necessary drugs in this world. There are so many drugs that are important to humanity now. The best situation would be collecting as many drugs as possible. However, give priority to those that are necessary.

Q. Which medical supplies should I give priority?

Priority should be given to regularly occurring conditions and conditions that affect your family. For instance, if you have a history of diabetes in your family, you may want to consider diabetes medication strongly. If someone in your family suffers from arthritis, it is important to get these drugs and other arthritis treatment supplies in bulk.

Besides the conditions available in your family, consider regularly occurring infections. Bacterial infections are very common. This means that you want to bring along as many antibiotics as possible. Make sure you stock antibiotics belonging to different classes and groups. I would not say stocking antivirals is necessary. Sometimes virus attacks are impossible to treat. MMO antivirals only work on specific viruses.

Also, make sure you bring along sufficient pain killers and some children's medication. This mix of products will go a long way in helping you serve your family and close relatives well in a situation of distress.

Q.Is it legal to stockpile medical supplies for the future?

Stoking medical supplies for the future is not legal in most areas. Civilians are only allowed to access medication through a prescription. Besides this, whatever you do is illegal.

Although you may find ways of collecting as many medical necessities as possible, your actions could land you in trouble unless you are discrete. You are required to only purchase drugs that you need based on a prescription. Any other action might be termed as drug abuse and may lead you to much trouble.

Q. What should I do with expired medication?

When you are stocking your prepper's pantry, remember that some of the substances you are stocking will expire. As a matter of fact, most drugs will expire before you get a chance to use them. This means that you should have a plan on how to deal with these substances as they expire.

One of the best strategies is to always ensure that what you stock is organized in such a way that expiration dates come gradually. Do not stock products that will expire on the same date closely. That is why I highly recommend gradual shopping. Make sure that for every drug type, you have different expiration periods. This way, you will only have to discard the drugs that have expired and replace them.

Q. Who should be given priority in severe critical cases?

As we have seen in the text above, priority should always be given to the most critical patient. This is followed by patients with special needs and then the rest. However, it is also in your best judgment to decide who to serve first. As mentioned, the main aim of a medical practitioner is to save as many lives as possible. In an SHFT event, you may have plenty of critically ill patients. In this case, you are required to start by serving the patient with chances of recovery. Do not go on wasting resources on a patient who may not recover entirely.

Q. How do you deal with mental health in an SHFT situation?

When all hell breaks loose, most people will suffer from mental and emotional problems. The situation you are in at the time will determine whether you will ever be in a position to use the medical supplies you have stocked up. It is important you have a way of dealing with your mental health. You must find healthy ways of releasing your emotions to avoid a situation where you end up getting mentally confused and unable to help even your closest family members.

Q. Can I perform surgery in an SHFT situation?

When there are no hospitals or anyone to help you get well, the possibilities of what you can do are endless. We have talked about amputations and why you should be able to carry out one in case you are in a bad place. It is necessary that you are in a position to perform an amputation and other surgeries when the need arises.

Conclusion

Preparing yourself medically for a dark day is important. Everyone should have at least some basic knowledge of health provision. Even if you are not interested in being a medical expert, you should at least have skills you can use in case you find yourself in a fix. These skills and medical supplies will come in handy where there are no doctors. You may use your skills to save a life.

In anticipation of such a dark day, it is also vital that you have medical references. You may download these medical documents from online sources. You also want to go to a bookshop and buy some books that will provide basic guidance on medical procedures. This way, you have knowledge of what you are doing in case you are in a doomsday situation.

Remember, you may not have power or access to the internet in an extreme emergency event, so be sure you have books on hand.

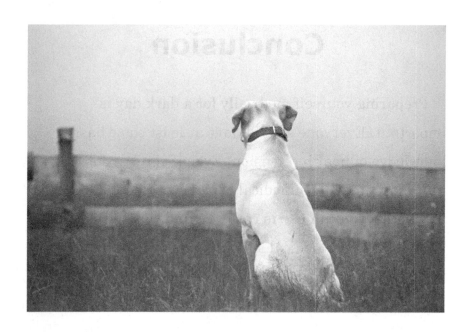

But before that day, please leave a review online where you purchased this book. I plan on reading all of the reviews so I can improve my next writing project.

Thanks in advance.

Made in the USA
Middletown, DE
29 October 2023

41576352R00096